Grief Diaries

SURVIVING LOSS OF HEALTH

True stories about coping with and managing lifelong health conditions

LYNDA CHELDELIN FELL
with
LAYNE MARTIN, R.N.
STACY ROORDA

FOREWORD BY LAYNE MARTIN, R.N.

Grief Diaries
Surviving Loss of Health – 1ˢᵗ ed.
True stories about coping with and managing lifelong health conditions
Lynda Cheldelin Fell/Layne Martin/Stacy Roorda
Grief Diaries www.GriefDiaries.com

Cover Design by AlyBlue Media, LLC
Interior Design by AlyBlue Media LLC
Published by AlyBlue Media, LLC

ISBN: 978-1-944328-08-5
AlyBlue Media, LLC
Ferndale, WA 98248
www.AlyBlueMedia.com

This book is designed to provide informative narrations to readers. It is sold with the understanding that the writers or publisher is not engaged to render any type of psychological, legal, or any other kind of professional advice. The content is the sole expression and opinion of the authors and writers. No warranties or guarantees are expressed or implied by the choice to include any of the content in this book. Neither the publisher nor the author or writers shall be liable for any physical, psychological, emotional, financial, or commercial damages including but not limited to special, incidental, consequential or other damages. Our views and rights are the same: You are responsible for your own choices, actions and results.

PRINTED IN THE UNITED STATES OF AMERICA

GRIEF DIARIES

TESTIMONIALS

"CRITICALLY IMPORTANT . . . *I want to say to Lynda that what you are doing is so critically important.*"
–DR. BERNICE A. KING, Daughter of Dr. Martin Luther King

"INSPIRATIONAL . . . *Grief Diaries: Loss by Impaired Driving is the result of heartfelt testimonials from a dedicated and loving group of people. By sharing their stories, the reader will learn the true devastation that impaired driving causes, and perhaps find inspiration and a renewed sense of comfort as they move through their own journey.*" -CANDACE LIGHTNER, Founder of Mothers Against Drunk Driving

"DEEPLY INTIMATE . . . *Loss of a Parent is a deeply intimate, authentic collection of narratives that speak to the powerful, often ambiguous, and wide spectrum of emotions that arise from the loss of one's mother or father. I so appreciate the vulnerability and truth embedded in these stories, which honor and bear witness to the many forms of bereavement that arise in the aftermath of parental death.*"
-DR. ERICA GOLDBLATT HYATT, Chair of Psychology, Bryn Athyn College

"MOVING . . . *We learn from stories throughout life. In Grief Diaries: Loss of a Parent the stories are not only moving but often provide a rich background for any mourner to find a gem of insight that can be used in coping with loss. Reread each story with pen in hand and you will find many that are just right for you.*" -DR. LOUIS LAGRAND, Author of Healing Grief, Finding Peace

"STUNNING . . . *Grief Diaries treats the reader to a rare combination of candor and fragility through the eyes of the bereaved. Delving into the deepest recesses of the heartbroken, the reader easily identifies with the diverse collection of stories and richly colored threads of profound love that create a stunning read full of comfort and hope.*" -DR. GLORIA HORSLEY, President of Open to Hope Foundation

"WONDERFUL . . . *Loss of a Sibling is a wonderful computation of stories written by the best of experts, bereaved siblings' themselves. Although this bond is one of life's longest and most unique relationships, sibling loss is often minimized and unacknowledged. Thank you for building awareness about a topic so near and dear to my heart.*" -DR. HEIDI HORSLEY, Adjunct Professor, School of Social Work, Columbia University, Grief Expert, Author, and Co-Founder of Open to Hope Organization

"CAPTIVATING . . . *Grieving for the Living is an inside look at the secret feelings we all experience as we navigate fragile relationships. The narrations are captivating, and will surely resonate deep within the hearts of those who face similar challenges.*" -DEANA L. MARTIN, Certified Grief Coach, Author, & Vice President of Cry for Me, No More

"HOPE AND HEALING . . . *You are a pioneer in this field and you are breaking the trail for others to find hope and healing.*"
-KRISTI SMITH, Bestselling Author & International Speaker

"INCREDIBLE . . . *Thank you so much for doing this project. it's absolutely incredible!*" -JULIE MJELVE, Founder, Grieving Together

"A FORCE . . . *The writers of this project, the Grief Diaries anthology series, are a force to be reckoned with. I'm betting we will be agents of great change.*"
-MARY LEE ROBINSON, Author and Founder of Set an Extra Plate initiative

"GLOBAL . . . *One of The Five Facets of Healing mantras is together we can heal a world of hurt. This anthology series is testimony to the power we have as global neighbors to do just that.*"
-ANNAH ELIZABETH, Founder of The Five Facets of Healing

"REWARDING . . . *This experience has been very rewarding for me. Just being able to talk with others who have walked this road.*" MONICA MIRKES, Grief Diaries writer

"SUPPORTED . . . *The project was very organized. The expectations were clear. The secret groups kept us all informed, and is where we all supported one another. I must say that I have been a part of very few things that were run this well! I have already signed up to be a part of one of the books in the next batch. And I look forward to being a part of that and any books that I qualify to be a part of in the future.*" -CHRISTINE BASTONE, author and writer

SURVIVING LOSS OF HEALTH

DEDICATION

This book is dedicated to the courageous writers who penned their intimate stories for the purpose of offering company, comfort and hope to others.

Christine Bastone
Jered Detwiler
Bonnie Forshey
Brenda Kleinsasser
Vicki Heckroth
Marlise Magna
Deana Martin
Layne Martin
Denise Purcell
MaryEllen Roach
Stacy Roorda
Lauren Vandal
Dawn Woinovick

SURVIVING LOSS OF HEALTH

CONTENTS

BY LAYNE MARTIN, R.N.

FOREWORD

Health is something we all cherish but tend to take for granted. We may get the occasional cold or seasonal flu that puts us out of commission for a few days, but when it passes and we start to feel well again, we're relieved to go on with daily life. Some people are more diligent about caring for their health, and protect it with regular exercise, eating a balanced diet, limiting alcohol use and avoiding smoking.

And then there are people like me who once had a healthy life before getting thrown into the abyss of the unknown when a significant health issue stops us in our tracks. Whether suddenly or gradually, the landscape shifts from our once-familiar routine to countless doctor appointments, lab tests, and uncomfortable procedures. Our entire world changes, and the loss of control can be frightening.

As it is with any loss, we find ourselves navigating stages of grief. And it can be a long, hard road. Our physical health, mental health, and social well-being become intertwined when our health declines, and we find ourselves longing for our old, familiar and comfortable routine. Sometimes the illness goes into remission or remains stable, and the person lives a fairly healthy life. Sometimes it doesn't and we're forced to rearrange life as we know it.

Grief Diaries has put together a compilation of stories from people all over the world who have experienced the loss of health firsthand. Our collective vision is to provide insight into the struggles faced by those suffering health challenges, and to offer their loved ones and caregivers some understanding which can lead to compassion and improved support.

Most importantly, our collective stories help those facing loss of health feel less alone as they begin their own navigation along this rocky path. For no matter where one is on this journey, we all share the same struggles, and there is some comfort in knowing we are not alone.

Layne Martin, R.N.
Blogger, Creaky Joints
www.CreakyJoints.com

PREFACE

One night in 2007, I had one of *those* dreams, the vivid kind you can't shake. In the dream, I was the front passenger in a car and my daughter Aly was sitting behind the driver. Suddenly, the car missed a curve in the road and sailed into a lake. The driver and I escaped the sinking car, but Aly did not. Desperately flailing through the deep murky water to find my daughter, I failed. She was gone. Aly was gone. The only evidence left behind was an open book floating face down on the water where my beloved daughter disappeared.

Two years later that nightmare became reality when my daughter, my third-born child, died as a back seat passenger in a car accident on August 5, 2009. She was just fifteen years old.

I now understand that the dream two years before Aly's death was a glimpse into a divine plan that would eventually touch many lives. The book left floating on the water was actually a peek at my future. But the devastation I felt in my heart would blind me to the meaning of that dream for a long time to come.

In the aftermath of losing Aly, I eventually discovered that helping others was a powerful way to heal my own heart. To my mind, one broken soul extending compassion to another in need is the ultimate act of human kindness. The Grief Diaries series was born and built on this belief.

By writing books that share our journeys through hardship and losses, our written words become a portable support group for others. When we swap stories, we feel less alone. It is comforting to know someone else understands the shoes we walk in, and the challenges we face along the way.

Which brings us to this book, *Grief Diaries: Surviving Loss of Health*. The devastation left in the aftermath of a lifelong health diagnosis can steal your breath, and leave you with more questions than answers. Further, you might encounter people who don't understand your emotions or, worse, lack compassion for your journey. This is where the *Grief Diaries* series can help.

Helen Keller once said, "Walking with a friend in the dark is better than walking alone in the light." This is especially true in the aftermath of any kind of loss. If you live with lifelong health challenges, the following true stories are written by courageous people who know exactly how you feel, for they've been in your shoes and have walked the same path. Perhaps the shoes are a different size or style, but may you find comfort in these stories and the understanding that you aren't truly alone on the journey. For we walk ahead, behind, and right beside you.

Wishing you healing, and hope from the Grief Diaries village.

Warm regards,

Warm regards,

Lynda Cheldelin Fell
Creator, Grief Diaries

CHAPTER ONE

THE BEGINNING

There is a plan and a purpose, a value to every life, no
matter what its location, age, gender or disability.
-SHARRON ANGLE

Health challenges are as unique to each individual as one's
fingerprint. In order to fully appreciate the different perspectives,
it is helpful to understand the different journeys. In this chapter,
each writer shares that moment when he or she was diagnosed with
an illness that would alter their entire future.

*

CHRISTINE BASTONE
Christine became ill with chronic
fatigue syndrome at the age of 27

In November 1993, I was at work on a temporary assignment
when all of a sudden I felt horrible. I don't remember what time it
was, except that it was morning. But one minute I was fine, and the
next minute I was not. I immediately got permission to go home.
There was no debating with myself about whether I should stay or
not. I originally thought it was a bad case of the flu, but I was never
the same after that. One of the first symptoms that I noticed was

1

feeling like all my energy flowed out of my body while I was taking a bath. Other symptoms included a frequent sore throat, a level of exhaustion that I had never before experienced, weakness in both my arms and legs, and brain fog. Pretty soon I was going to the doctor numerous times, but he kept telling me I was just depressed. Of course I was depressed, I felt absolutely awful every day! On my own, I did some researching at the library, and ultimately I was the one who figured out that what I had was chronic fatigue syndrome. My biggest clue was that exercising brought on my symptoms, and made me feel like I had been hit by a truck. But I couldn't get anyone else to believe me. At the time people just didn't "believe" in this disease, and that included doctors. I think that very slowly belief is growing, but, even so, many people still don't believe in it. I have pretty much been on my own dealing with this illness. And I can't tell you how lonely that is, or how absolutely invalidating all the disbelief that I have run into has been.

In order to get to the part where I tell you how I got my diagnosis, you have to fast forward about eight years. It took me about this long to figure out that every cycle of push, push, push until I crashed, only to start pushing again, made me weaker each time. Oh, how I wish that I had figured that out a lot sooner. I am sure that I would be feeling a lot better than I do, and also be able to do more things.

I basically have three levels of how I feel with this illness. The first one is feeling like I've been hit by a truck. I feel this way most of the time. Second, there is a feeling like death warmed over. Thankfully I don't feel this way quite as often. But it's still an all too familiar feeling. Third is like a stretched out rubber band. Feeling this was what made me realize that I was getting weaker with each cycle. This level is the worst. I can't read, I can't watch TV, I can't even rest comfortably. All I can do is wait for this feeling to go away, and then do anything I can to avoid feeling this level again. I've done pretty well with this third level, as I can count on one hand the number of times I have felt this way.

By the time eight years had passed I was married, had an infant son, and was working in the evenings part-time. I quit that job shortly after I got my diagnosis. But before I did that, I wrote a letter to my new doctor and described what I thought I had, and asked him to help me. He basically just took a blood test. When he told me the results, he said that I was right because it showed up that I had the Epstein-Barr virus. But he said that the only thing I could do for it was to take Prozac. While I have never agreed with him about that, I was very relieved to finally get a diagnosis.

*

JERED DETWILER
Jered was diagnosed with a rare liver disorder,
Glycogen Storage Disease type 1a, as an infant
and hepatocellular cancer with liver tumors at age 31

I was born with a rare genetic condition called Glycogen Storage Disease 1a. When I was born no one knew I had it. The symptoms are chronic low blood sugar and an enlarged liver. As a baby my mom took me to the doctor for a checkup and the doctor noticed my liver was enlarged. I was sent to the hospital to have many tests to figure out what the problem was. It took about a month for them to figure it out and even then the doctors were unsure of the type of Glycogen Storage Disease I had as there are several types. But they guessed it was type 1a, which mainly affects the liver. One process of the liver is to store glycogen to use when the blood sugar begins to drop. In my liver there is no door to let the stores of glycogen out to raise the blood sugar when it drops so the glycogen continually stores and enlarges my liver.

There is no cure yet for Glycogen Storage Disease, or GSD as we call it. The only treatment is to keep the blood sugar up. Since my body can't keep the blood sugar up on its own I have to eat a complex carbohydrate every four to six hours. I eat a lot of crackers, cereal and rice. I also drink a few tablespoons of uncooked cornstarch in a glass of water in the morning. As the cornstarch

3

digests it turns to glucose slowly and enters my system to help keep my blood sugar up for several hours at a time. I have had to drink cornstarch in water all my life to help keep my blood sugar up.

Living with GSD has its ups and downs. For instance my blood sugar might go low if I don't eat on time, or when I get sick. When it goes low I usually get shaky and sometimes I get a headache or just feel rotten. My mom can see it on my face, my lips turn ashen and my skin feels cold and clammy.

One of the other medical problems that the GSD has caused is a condition called gout. Most people get it in their toe, I have it in my knee and my ankle. As a baby my knee was swollen and when my mom took me to the doctor to figure out what the problem was I was diagnosed with gout. This was the only flair up I had as a child. However, with my liver not working correctly the gout has been an ongoing challenge in adulthood. It causes my knee or my ankle to fill with fluid. It is very painful and I have had the fluid drawn out of my knee on several occasions. During the flares, I have difficulty walking and sometimes use a cane. It can be strange to see a young adult using a cane. I do take medication daily to help keep the gout in check.

As a teen my liver began to grow little tumors called adenomas. This is also common for a person who has GSD 1a. The adenomas are not a problem usually and I don't feel any different with them on my liver. Since they grow slowly it can be many years before they change to anything more than just a little fatty tumor. However they can change to cancer. The tumors on my liver began to change last year and I was sent to a liver tumor clinic at the local university. I was sent for scans and then returned to the clinic every few months so they could follow the growth of the tumors for changes. As the tumors began to change, the doctor suggested I have a biopsy of one of the tumors. The biopsy revealed that I had small hepatocellular cancer cells in the tumor. Now I have to live with life-threatening cancer. The only cure is to have the tumors removed surgically or to have a liver transplant. Surgically removing the tumors was discussed but I have a set of twin tumors that surround a major vessel in my liver. I was told that it was too dangerous to try to remove the tumors, and the doctors just didn't think they could remove all the tumors which meant the cancer could still grow. So my only opportunity at health would be to have a liver transplant. I was sent to the transplant clinic at the university. I go for regular appointments while I wait for a liver transplant. Each time I go in, I have bloodwork done and have an MRI of my liver so the tumors can be checked for growth. The doctors talk to me after the tests and then I go home. Each person on the transplant list has a transplant score, called a MELD score which stands for "model for end-stage liver disease." The MELD score is raised every few months when I go in for my clinic appointments. A score of 30 is about the top of the list. My score today is 28 and now I'm just waiting for a transplant. While I wait, I cannot go anywhere that is very far away to ensure that I can get to the hospital within a two-hour window. I don't mind not going very far away now. It will be totally worth it.

*

BONNIE FORSHEY
Bonnie was diagnosed with hepatitis C at age 41, rheumatoid and osteoarthritis at age 48, diabetes and systemic lupus at age 50, and Graves' disease and MAC disease at age 60

The loss of my health all began when I was a student nurse. I was working in the medical-surgical unit and had been assigned a new patient. This was in the 1980s, when we didn't know much about hepatitis C. I went in to assess the patient and noticed that he was very jaundiced. Before I knew what was happening, he became ill and vomited blood which totally saturated me. The patient was taken to surgery and I had to go to the physician's lounge to shower and discard my scrubs. I wrote up an incident report and tried to forget about it. But the ugly truth surfaced in 1993 when I was diagnosed with hepatitis C, and I have been battling it ever since.

I have become very ill over the years, and have developed many other comorbidities as a result of the hepatitis C. I have been diagnosed with systemic lupus, rheumatoid arthritis, osteoarthritis, diabetes type II, gastroparesis, gastro reflux, Graves' disease, asthma, chronic heart failure, Raynaud's disease, depression, and mycobacterial avium complex. I have chronic pain and have an indwelling pain pump so I don't have to take oral pain medications, but it only covers the lumbar spine area.

I was treated for the hepatitis C during the beginning of 2015. I took the treatment for twelve weeks, and the virus was undetected. I felt wonderful, my energy returned, my other illnesses went into remission, and I enjoyed quality time with my grandsons and daughter. It was wonderful. I haven't been able to work since 2005, and it felt like a new beginning.

About seven months after treatment I began to feel ill again. I went in for bloodwork and it was determined that the virus had indeed reared its ugly little head again. My physician wanted to find out why I had relapsed and ordered more tests. My liver had stage IV cirrhosis caused by the virus. Now I know why it is deemed, "The Silent Killer." It starts to destroy your liver before you even know that you have it. That's why everyone should get checked for it, before it's too late. Needless to say, I was devastated. I feel like someone is dangling a carrot in front of my face and no matter what I do, I can't reach it. I had a brief period of happiness and now it is gone, just like a bad dream. The news made me fall into a deep depression and I just wanted to give up. I went to see my hepatologist (liver doctor) and we discussed other options. She was ready to start me on another treatment but she first had to talk it over with the department head, to get his approval. I was very excited and began to gear myself up mentally for another battle. A week later my liver doctor called and told me that the department head wanted me to be in a study at the hospital. He denied me the treatment, and I was crushed again. I emailed my liver doctor, and she said the study would be in six months.

I have been going through pure hell for thirty-five years. I made up my mind that I was not waiting for any study and that I would not take no for an answer. I called her office repeatedly, every day. I called her cell phone. I sent text messages and emails. I was on a mission and had to become proactive. This was my life, my health, and the clock was ticking. Eventually, they became sick of my constant presence in their everyday routines. The department head finally agreed upon a new treatment and I would soon be in another battle to rid myself of HCV. I have just begun a new treatment with Viekira, a new antiviral medication, and I will be on it for twelve weeks. I started it in August after having to wait for my physician to get the okay from my insurance company. I am in another battle and pray that I get rid of this virus.

More than likely, I will be looking to have a liver transplant in the future, but I can handle anything that life puts in my path. Being chronically ill has made me a very strong and determined woman. I have been put in a real dilemma, as my other illnesses can't be treated until my liver is taken care of. All of the drugs that I need are so toxic to the liver.

I suffer with severe joint pain all of the time, but at least I am alive, and there is always hope. The rheumatoid arthritis and lupus have taken a toll on my body. I have severe joint pain and can do very little for myself. I was always so independent and did everything for myself, now I can't even fasten my own buttons or do any of the things that used to give me pleasure, such as gardening, sewing and crafts. I stay tired all of the time, it is difficult to use my hands, and difficult to walk.

Patient care was my passion and I will never be able to return to nursing. I was a very strong and fiercely independent woman. I raised two children alone, put myself through college and nursing school while working a full-time job, and maintained my own home and yard maintenance. It is gut wrenching to be reduced to such a weak individual, to have to depend on others, and become a person that is almost unrecognizable to me when I gaze into the mirror. I also have mycobacterium avium complex (MAC) disease of the lungs and asthma. I have a difficult time breathing and I cough all of the time. The least little thing wears me out and places me in jeopardy.

It's the little things in life that we take for granted. I am not happy with the way that my life has played out. It has been a very difficult journey, but it is mine. I have to accept it and deal with it. I am still alive, so there is always hope. Five years ago there was no hope for chronic hepatitis C. Now I am on my way to being cured. Maybe there will be a cure for my other autoimmune diseases, as well. That strong, independent woman is hidden in there somewhere, and she helps me to remain hopeful and to stay strong.

*

VICKI HECKROTH
Vicki was diagnosed with rheumatoid
arthritis and fibromyalgia at age 45

My health deteriorated very quickly after the loss of my seventeen-year-old son Matt to suicide in 2000. They tell me it was heightened due to the stress I was under. One day I was fine, the next I was a little stiff but credited it to working fifteen-hour shifts as the manager of Burger King. However within three days the pain was so bad that I could barely walk. I went from a walker to a wheelchair to an electric chair rather quickly. I went to doctor after doctor until finally being diagnosed with rapidly progressing seronegative rheumatoid arthritis and fibromyalgia. Thanks to medication to help stop the progression and also high potent pain medication, I am now able to walk on my own and function at a level where at least I feel like I am living.

*

BRENDA L. KLEINSASSER
Brenda was diagnosed with rheumatoid arthritis at age 31
and a right frontal lobe meningioma brain tumor at age 48

I had no idea when I bumped my head inside that fridge, over seven years ago, that my life would change forever. Not at first anyway. I thought I was just careless when I put my head in too far and bumped it on the switch, which really hurt, and so I thought that I just bruised it good. I didn't get knocked out, so I thought why go to a doctor? Not good advice to ignore any head injury EVER! Well it hurt for a while and got better, so I thought everything would be fine.

Months later though, it really started to hurt, so I went to my doctor. He said I probably just bruised it bad and it would just take some time to heal. Well, it got better and then it got worse. I had a skull x-ray and it showed nothing. My doctor put me on something for pain and a sedative so I could sleep. I had to stop taking the pain medication because I started having muscle aches.

It got better over time again, so I thought it was just badly bruised and would take time to heal. By August 2007, just after my father passed away from Alzheimer's, I went to see a neurologist who said it was a pulled muscle. He recommended exercises and felt this would help it get better. He also said we could do a CT scan but we would more than likely not find anything. So believing in my doctor, I did nothing other than to go home and do the exercises. Little did I know at this point that there was something actually WRONG! I went home and like a good patient, started doing the exercises and it did seem to get better, so I thought, maybe they were right about the pulled muscle.

By spring 2008, it was getting much worse. I was starting to feel like something was really active in there, but you know how the brain works. When you feel it on one side the culprit is actually on the opposite side. I really did not know anything conclusive at this point.

By summer, I just could not take it anymore. I asked my doctor's nurse if I could have a CT scan. She called me on the phone and, this still makes me angry when I think about it, said not once, but twice in our telephone conversation that if we find nothing on the scan then we are done. She asked me if I understood her statement. Well, I just knew they would have to find something.

In August 2008, I had the head CT scan. Lo and behold, they found a lesion on the right frontal lobe of my brain. I was not crazy after all! The next step was to schedule an MRI for that same week. I thought, now I will finally have my answer. WRONG! I went to the hospital for the MRI and they asked me if I was claustrophobic. I really didn't know, but BELIEVE ME, I knew after six minutes that YES, I was claustrophobic. I told them I had to get out of there. They said they could reschedule under anesthesia but had to schedule it for another day. I was devastated. I just couldn't believe I couldn't handle the MRI. I had been through so much already!

The MRI was rescheduled for the following week, and I had no trouble other than being really sick afterward. I got home that night and there was a message on my answering machine from my doctor. So I called, but he was having dinner and his wife asked if he could call me back. I said that would be fine. When my doctor called back, he said I had what is called a meningioma, no larger than a walnut, but that it could be monitored for now. Now, I wanted that thing out of my head yesterday! My doctor said to call his office the next day, and they would schedule an appointment with a neurologist. If the neurologist felt a neurosurgeon was necessary, they would go from there. I was not excited about seeing that same neurologist again. You see, to him everything is a joke. This was no joke to me. I didn't know it at the time, but it was an actual brain tumor. I was in shock!

I had to wait another week, the longest week of my entire life. My mother accompanied me on that visit, and when we were taken back to the exam room, the nurse asked a few questions. The neurologist then entered the room, and I have to tell it to you straight folks, it did not look good. He said the tumor had probably had been there for over twenty years, but the other pain I felt in my head was not the cause. Maybe so, but that original pain alerted me to ask for the CT in the first place. My point is this: YOU know when something is WRONG with your body. Don't EVER be afraid to ask for any tests!

The examination went on. The doctor showed me the mass, it now looked like the shape of an egg. I really had no idea how large it was at this point. The doctor finally asked if I wanted to see a neurosurgeon. Just like that, things started to turn in our favor. I said yes. He asked if I wanted to see one today, again I said yes. He walked me down the hall to the neurosurgeon. When his nursing assistant walked in the room, I instantly liked her. She was so understanding. She said that the neurosurgeon would be right in. He walked in and showed me the tumor in depth, contrast and noncontrast. He asked if I wanted it out, stating that he wouldn't know anything concrete until it was examined under a microscope. I of course said YES! That was Thursday, September 4, 2008. Another CT was performed and the surgery, a craniotomy, was scheduled for Monday, September 8. That was the day when my second chance began.

My surgery was expected to be about two hours, but took only ninety minutes as the tumor was solid and very easy to get at. It measured just a bit smaller than a golf ball. It was located in the right frontal lobe. The doctor told my mother it was marble size, but quickly corrected himself.

WOW, so that is how it all began. If I would never have bumped my head in that fridge, I probably would still have this tumor and it would have headed right toward my motor skills. At least that's what the neurosurgeon said.

I also have lived with rheumatoid arthritis (RA) for over twenty-four years. When I finally received a copy of my MRI, things really started to make sense. It mentioned that my sinuses were involved, so that would explain the many nosebleeds I experienced, which I found out later, could actually be a sign of a brain tumor. Also there was something there that mimicked multiple sclerosis, MS, which also made sense because of the rheumatoid arthritis. My life truly changed from that whole experience.

*

MARLISE MAGNA
Marlise was diagnosed with epilepsy in 1996, fibromyalgia and insulin resistance in 2009, and posttraumatic stress disorder in 2014

My first loss of health started in 1996 with the diagnosis of temporal lobe epilepsy. I was seventeen and in my final school year but the symptoms started when I was around ten years-old. I will never forget the time I had my first symptom. My brother and I were at a restaurant for supper with my dad and his girlfriend. I remember suddenly getting this intense migraine-like headache and being so nauseous and unable to look at lights. I laid on my dad's lap and recall hearing him say to his girlfriend, "I hope this isn't epilepsy." Even at that age I remember wondering to myself how he made the jump from a headache to epilepsy, though both my parents majored in psychology at university so it wasn't unusual for them to think outside the box.

As the years progressed I continually suffered severe migraines and later on started having olfactory hallucinations, smelling odd things like copper, blood and burning wires. I also started seeing movements from the corners of my eyes. Eventually after many tests and visits to neurologists, I got my diagnosis.

That started me on a long and hard road. At one point I was taking thirty-three anti-epilepsy pills each day. There's about two years of my life I simply cannot recall due to being so drugged up and sleeping continually. I barely ate yet I gained a huge amount of weight due to the medication. Which led to my next health issue, being insulin resistant.

Matters weren't helped when in 2007 out of sheer desperation and being pre-diabetic, I opted to have Roux-en-Y gastric bypass surgery. For the record, please let me state that even though this option does work, it is not a quick fix and the aftereffects are lifelong and very severe - malnutrition, fatigue, lowered immune system, etc. The surgeon who pioneered this operation himself said years later that he probably should not have messed with God's creation.

After the bypass I was chronically ill and almost died from lack of potassium and iron. I developed fibromyalgia, and I've heard that major surgery or a severe shock can cause that. I was at my doctor's office at least once a week. He finally figured out it might be fibromyalgia and referred me to a rheumatologist. Sadly, none of the prescribed medications had any effect so it's still an ongoing battle managing chronic and sometimes debilitating pain.

My posttraumatic stress disorder was diagnosed in 2014. I'd been through an extremely rough breakup with my boyfriend, had two failed marriages, and lost my partner to suicide. I guess my mind could only take so much.

That said, I regret nothing. Everything that has happened has made me a stronger person. I am a survivor, not a victim, and that's what makes me a force to be reckoned with!

*

DEANA MARTIN
Deana was diagnosed with chronic depression and anxiety disorder at age 26, breast cancer at age 33, and posttraumatic stress disorder at age 45 after losing both children in a car accident

To lose health one must first have health. I can't say that I have ever truly been what one would call healthy. All my bloodwork and medical tests normally come back either outstanding or with minimal issues. However I have always been overweight, even as a child. I was diagnosed with chronic depression and anxiety disorder in 1991, at the age of twenty-six. The professionals who diagnosed this while I was in an outpatient mental health treatment facility believe that, due to patterns in my life, there is a likelihood that I have been dealing with mental health issues all my life that went undiagnosed as a child. I suffered from learning disabilities which the anxiety and depression only exacerbated and vice versa. Whenever I faced a great deal of stress the dyslexia would become a huge issue, continuing to jeopardize my career again and again. Management does not take kindly to repeated errors in spelling and math, let alone transposing numbers.

As a young woman I dealt with various health issues that were not common for my age such as bursitis, sciatica, irritable bowel syndrome and gallbladder attacks just to name a few. I mentioned in Grief Diaries: Grieving for the Living that I discovered early on that illness at least got me some attention that I always sought from my family. I became a mother at age twenty, still a child myself. As a mother and caretaker of a family there is no time for illness. The children, house and husband come first and I became a codependent caretaker. The majority of my health issues went out the window along with what felt like the minimal sanity I had most days. I still experienced problems with irritable bowel syndrome and my gallbladder but I tried to either ignore it or not let it keep me down long because there were floors to clean and laundry to be done.

At age thirty-three, after working in a chemistry lab around carcinogenic agents for one of the fortune 500 pharmaceutical companies, I developed breast cancer. Breast cancer does not run in my family and I had no doubt that it was the poor air handling and exposure to these lethal chemicals that caused my cells to rebel against me. I was just starting to dabble into eastern medicine and other healing modalities at the time and from my mystical brain I was convinced that since the cancer was in my left (female) breast (mothering), it was brought on symbolically by my resentment of my mother and of being a mother. I struggled with a great portion of my life, which I wrote about in Grief Diaries: Grieving for the Living. This experience with cancer was the first time I had to face my own mortality and, to put it simply, was scared sh**less. My babies were young, early teen and preteen, and I begged God to let me live to see them graduate high school. When I found out I had breast cancer, I had just spent five years piecing my shattered family back together after it was revealed that my third husband had molested my daughter. I followed the advice of the mental health professionals, and went through all the steps to put my family back together and ensure that the children and both my husband and I received the healing that was needed. I never understood why they told me that treatment and putting our "Brady Bunch" family back together was so important, but I went along with it knowing the therapy could not hurt. Then it dawned on me one day that if I told the courts to lock up my husband and throw away the key, that my daughter and our other children would be learning hate, vengeance, and that if a person in our society screwed up bad enough they would simply be thrown away.

This was when I was able to see the big picture, that this treatment we were advised to seek helped everyone to learn love, forgiveness, and that people sometimes make huge mistakes but that does not mean the person is bad, rather that the action, as it was in our case, was caused by mental illness. We learned that people can heal and that the capacity of the human heart to love is greater than hatred.

When I was diagnosed with breast cancer, after trying to keep everyone afloat for five years and therapy for someone in our little clan every night of the week, my husband could not deal with my fears of death due to losing his female primary caretaker at a young age (mother and maternal grandmother) which left him and his sister alone in the world. For me, that was the last straw. After all I had endured to ensure our family healed from the trauma he had caused, I no longer could continue to play that role, the role of compassion and love. We were physically together and he helped care for me through my treatment, but I could never again trust him, that he would be there for me as I had been for him.

My dance with the devil through surgery, chemo and radiation was a trauma that would linger for years, leaving me always fearful that it would return. Cancer was in my mind in the beginning each moment of the day, just as my children's death was eighteen years later when they left me for places unknown through a fatal car accident. That was when I realized that unresolved trauma and grief, along with posttraumatic stress disorder, had ruled a large portion of my life and to be very honest still does today. I imagine it always will too. I don't have the energy or the money to seek out every healing modality and treatment under the sun as I did years ago. At times, I simply wait for the next blow to my health or mental stability.

I have also suffered from suicidal ideation for years although I didn't know what it was when I was younger. So when asked to discuss the loss of my health and the events leading up to it, there was no cut and dry answer. My health both mental and physical have always been and continue to be a challenge that I am not sure I care much about these days. Since my beloved children left, I have my bags packed and I am ready to join them at any time. I now have a myriad of other health issues since their death, my body rebelled in ways I could never have imagined.

*

LAYNE MARTIN
Layne was diagnosed
with psoriatic arthritis at age 47

Having worked as a nurse most of my life, when my symptoms of psoriatic arthritis started I just chalked it up to long days and being on my feet for twelve-hour shifts. As my disease progressed it started a series of misdiagnosis by multiple doctors which delayed proper treatment and further damage to my joints.

Now that I look back, I know that my disease may have lay dormant in my body for many years and was triggered by a life altering event. That event was in 1999 when my husband came home one day and announced that he had quit his job as a teacher. Not only was I shocked, but our life as we knew it for the last fifteen years was turned upside down! For the sake of our children I put on a happy face and held strong as my husband uprooted us to move across state to his new teaching job.

As I got the kids settled and they started new schools, I started the hunt for a new job. I soon landed a job as the emergency department manager at a hospital in the greater Seattle area. It was a much larger hospital than I was used to working in, and I managed over one hundred employees.

Soon my first symptom of psoriatic arthritis started. It started with intense itching and flaking of my scalp. It became so bad that I started wearing only cream colored or pastel blouses and tops. And I had my hairdresser put blonde highlights in my brunette hair to help camouflage the flakes. After trying several different shampoos, I went to the doctor and she said it was just a bad case of dandruff and prescribed a steroid lotion.

Next my feet started to bother me. As a nurse manager, I had to wear business attire each day. Walking around the large hospital in my dress shoes was excruciating. After purchasing an endless variety of shoes and inserts, I went to see a podiatrist. He diagnosed my swollen "sausage toes" as Morton's neuroma. I now know that "sausage toes" are a classic sign of psoriatic arthritis. I was also having a terrible time with my right hip. I had been born with bilateral congenital hip dysplasia and spent the first year of my life in and out of a body cast. I sought the advice of my primary care doctor and after x-rays he determined that I had hip bursitis most likely caused from my career and long hours on my feet. That was the point when I began a series of cortisone hip injections every three to four months.

As my disease progressed I started having joint stiffness and low back pain. I went to my doctor and after some lab testing he said it was probably polymyalgia rheumatic and placed me on daily low-dose cortisone. I felt fairly well on the cortisone and continued working and raising my two busy active teenagers for the next eight years. But then my hip stopped responding to the cortisone injections, and an MRI revealed that I needed a total hip replacement at the age of forty-seven.

In between that time we moved again, back to the small town we had originally raised our children, and my husband started a new job as a school principal. I was now the nurse manager of not only an emergency department but also the medical-surgical unit, so I worked right up until the day before my surgery. It wasn't until after the surgery and the pathology came back on my hip that the doctors considered an autoimmune disease. I was finally referred to a rheumatologist where I was diagnosed with psoriatic arthritis. I was able to go back to work after eight weeks of rehabilitation. However, the many years of cortisone therapy took a toll on my body and I developed two compression fractures in my thoracic spine that cause excruciating pain. I struggled and fought the inevitable but, at age forty-nine, relented to my disease and retired from the profession I so dearly loved.

Retirement threw me into a very dark place as I struggled with my identity and sense of self-worth. I found comfort in vodka! I started my affair with vodka in 1999, when my world was initially turned upside down and I was uprooted from a place and house that I dearly loved. As the years progressed I never once thought it was a problem. After all, everyone had a cocktail or two when they got home from work. I told myself that I worked a stressful job so it was a nice way to unwind and relax at the end of the day. Besides, I never once called in sick because of it and it wasn't affecting my job performance so who cares. Once I was diagnosed with psoriatic arthritis then I really had a great excuse and told my doctors and physical therapist that I used it for medicinal purposes. That opened the door for lots of valid excuses and the drinks became taller and stronger. One doctor told me I should probably cut back a bit but dealing with my alcohol use really didn't seem to be a big concern so I continued to indulge and self-medicate, sending me on a rollercoaster ride that eventually came to a sudden stop.

Finding my sense of purpose and taking control of my health and my life was a long tough battle. I still battle every day but without the use of vodka. A lot of what I've learned has been trial and error but I love sharing my story and I hope I can reach out and help others by sharing what I've learned.

*

DENISE PURCELL
Denise was diagnosed with fibromyalgia
and degenerative disc disease at age 45

I started having flu like symptoms that would keep me in bed and unable to do things for weeks at a time. I could hardly stay awake past 7 p.m. Household chores were painful so I went to the doctor. She examined me and when she touched my pressure points, I screamed. That is how I found out about the fibromyalgia.

The degenerative disc disease was diagnosed in 2010. I had severe pain radiating down my arm which I thought was a pinched nerve. I was sent to an orthopedist doctor who gave me a cortisone injection, but it didn't help.

I then went for a mammogram and noticed that when I hung onto the machine handles, my neck hurt severely. I returned to the orthopedist, and this time they did an MRI which revealed bone spurs were narrowing my spinal canal and I also had degenerative disc disease. I underwent surgery and they went through the front of my neck to put in a plate and pin. They also went through the back of the neck to remove some of the bone spurs.

And then in 2013 my lower back showed signs of worsening disc disease. I underwent a lower laminectomy with bone graft and fusion, similar to my neck, but with a cage and hardware. Two months later, because the pain remained, they found out that a screw had been hitting a nerve, resulting in yet another surgery to fix that.

*

MARYELLEN ROACH
MaryEllen was diagnosed
with fibromyalgia at age 30

I don't remember exactly when my symptoms began, but I do remember being exhausted in high school and feeling the painful burning sensation in my back that I am now very familiar with. At the time I just thought I was tired because I got up so early for school, and the back pain was probably because I was overweight. The first time I remember experiencing excruciating pain from fibromyalgia, although I didn't know it was fibromyalgia at the time, was when I was twenty-seven. It was December in the Midwest which meant it was very cold with temperatures well below freezing. I had just parked and got out of my car at my workplace, picked up my bags and began the trek to the building. My back was hurting as usual, but the further I walked and the colder I got, I began feeling an overwhelming pain in my arms, shoulders, ribcage, chest and back, which made it hard to breathe. My eyes were almost to the point of watering because it hurt so badly. I had to stop a couple of times to breathe and give my body a few seconds to relax before walking again. When I finally made it inside the building and felt the warmth, the pain subsided and I went about my workday. The pain scared me because it had never been so intense, so I made an appointment with a doctor. The doctor told me that all the muscles in my torso were inflamed and she was prescribing an anti-inflammatory. The medication helped me get through the rest of the winter and life went on.

A few years later, my boyfriend at the time and I were joking around and he poked my arm with his finger. The pain was overwhelming and I was angry because I thought he had intentionally hurt me, so I asked why he did that. He responded that he didn't do it hard and it wouldn't hurt if I did the same to him, so I did. To my amazement, it didn't hurt him at all, but the pain in my arm was still radiating and it continued for about ten to fifteen minutes. That exchange was the first time I realized everyone didn't hurt the same way I always had. That same boyfriend would always joke with me about how I never sat still and one evening he bet me that I couldn't sit completely still for five minutes straight. Being the competitive person I am, I gladly accepted his challenge and planned to show him I could do it. However, after about two minutes, I felt the overwhelming urge to move and it was then that I realized I constantly moved because of pain. I still resisted the urge, but the pain became more and more intense until I simply could not keep from moving. As soon as I gave in and moved, the pain eased a bit and I felt some relief.

I made an appointment with another doctor and as I explained to her what had happened, she decided to refer me to a rheumatologist in her office. My blood was drawn and tested for lupus, multiple sclerosis, arthritis and other diseases. When I saw the doctor to find out the results, I was told all of those tests came back negative. I was relieved I didn't have any of those things, but then the rheumatologist pressed different pressure points around my body and most of them created that same radiating, burning pain I had felt before. She then told me that I was being diagnosed with fibromyalgia. I had heard that name before, but wasn't completely familiar with it. When I got home I looked it up online and was blown away by the description and symptoms because they fit what I had been experiencing for years. Some of the symptoms listed were anxiety, depression, chronic fatigue, widespread pain and achiness, stiffness, inability to concentrate and many others. One symptom in particular made me remember that December from a few years earlier: hypersensitivity to cold. I realized that the experience I had was called a fibro flare, where fibromyalgia had raised its ugly head and roared. The doctor prescribed Cymbalta which is actually an antidepressant, but it has also been found to help with fibromyalgia pain. I don't like taking medication, but I reluctantly accepted and began taking it as prescribed. After a couple of weeks I could tell a huge difference in how I felt and began to understand how "normal" people feel. Unfortunately the relief was short-lived as the medication stopped working after a couple of months. I decided at that time that I preferred to live life unmedicated and only take an over the counter pain reliever when I really needed to.

It has now been seven years since I was diagnosed and I am able to recognize how much fibromyalgia affects my life. I wake up exhausted every day not only because fatigue is a part of it, but also because I toss and turn a lot at night from the pain. Most of the time when I get out of bed I am very sore and stiff. The burning sensation in my back usually resumes as I brush my teeth at the bathroom sink. The pain never goes away; it's like a combination of living with the flu constantly and muscles feeling like I've worked out too hard. I still have to be extremely careful not to get too cold, otherwise I pay for it with more intense pain for several days afterward.

Stress and emotional upset also make the symptoms much worse. My forty-one-year-old sister Suzette and her two daughters, eight-year-old Lillian and six-year-old Vivian moved to heaven in July 2012 due to a car accident. Since losing the three of them and dealing with the life changes and seemingly endless pit of grief, I have struggled harder than ever. I have more flares now and some days I literally cannot stay awake. Simple things like cooking, cleaning, applying makeup, standing in one place to talk to someone, even just sitting on the floor and so many other things are difficult to do at times and sometimes impossible. When asked to do something, I am forced to base my decision on the pain value of the activity and decide if I can handle it or not. Recently I had to turn down a camping trip because although it would be so much fun, the pain would outweigh it. One of the biggest challenges has been admitting when I can't do something because of the fatigue or pain. It is embarrassing when I can't do what I want and especially activities with friends or family. Living with fibromyalgia is depressing at times and I just want to be like most people who can wake up and do whatever they want instead of letting pain decide what my day will be. It is a challenge every minute of every day, but I refuse to let it beat me. I may have it, but it doesn't have me.

*

STACY ROORDA
Stacy was diagnosed with
metastatic breast cancer at age 37

I was transitioning from a career woman to being a stay-at-home mom of two young daughters when we moved into a large, new home in my husband's small hometown. For six months I had slightly annoying arm pain but attributed the pestering symptoms to the strains of moving. Finally I went to see my naturopath in late November 2006, thinking it was nothing major. The naturopath, much to my shock, was immediately suspicious of something more sinister. She sent me for a battery of tests. The devastating results arrived the day before Thanksgiving: I had stage four breast cancer, and it was aggressive.

A potent treatment plan was formulated until two weeks later more bloodwork revealed a second shock that halted everything and tested my faith like nothing else: I was pregnant. Not only that but the cancer was feeding on the very hormone my body was producing in large amounts: estrogen. As I walked out of the clinic I asked God, "Lord what does this mean?" I immediately got an image of a four-point harness that race car drivers wear. The feeling was instant, "Sit down and buckle up. It's going to be a rough road, but you'll be fine." I grabbed onto that thought and never let go.

*

LAUREN VANDAL
Lauren suffered a traumatic
brain injury at age 35

I moved to Northern Ireland from West Yorkshire in 2012, on a whimsical notion of packing up and starting again. Up until then life was pretty much running fairly smoothly. I had a job, hobbies, friends and a husband. It was in 2012, when I decided I was bored with everything. I had that vague notion that there's more to life than this. So I ended my marriage, quit my job and decided to move across the sea. Shortly after moving to Northern Ireland I joined the local roller derby team. I used to play in England and it was one of the things that had saved my sanity on many occasion! I was excited to make connections here and continue playing the sport I loved. Then, the accident happened, and my life would change dramatically. I was at a training session one afternoon when I made physical contact at speed with another person. This was all part of the sport, so nothing unusual. But I hit my head and something felt like it snapped in my head. I knelt on the floor and soon realized I couldn't see my hands in front of my face. In fact, I couldn't see anything. Everything went dark and that's when the old Lauren died.

I came around five days later in the ICU ward in Belfast. I had absolutely no idea where I was or why. My family had flown over from England and my partner had been sitting by my side every day. My first thought was how hungry I was, my second thought was when could I go home? It turns out I had suffered a subdural hematoma. Following a CT scan at the hospital, I underwent emergency brain surgery to relieve the pressure in my skull and save my life. I had a craniotomy and woke with half my hair missing, various tubes hanging out of me and a rather impressive scar. My loss was sudden and unexpected and, for a long time, very misunderstood. I had no idea of the journey about to unfold.

*

DAWN WOINOVICK
Dawn was diagnosed with depression, posttraumatic stress disorder, degenerative disc disease at age 37, and a pituitary tumor at age 52

I suffer from PTSD, depression, and major anxiety from extensive incest and other abuse. And I have been disabled since about 2000, due to degenerative disc disease. One disc was gone and a second one was in sad shape. I spent eighteen months learning how to live with my broken body and pain. It took the doctors a few years to get the pain under control. A morphine patch helped but "no pain, no brain." I lost a lot of what was me. I gained forty pounds and lost my teeth. I finally got a doctor to help me get off the morphine and to help me clear my head. To look at me you would not have known I was disabled. Until now.

By October 2014, I was having mega migraines, a hard time seeing, I was gaining weight and leaking breast milk even though I had a partial hysterectomy. My equilibrium was off, I was falling down a lot, I had no depth perception. When you're a kid, it's funny to see someone walk into a door or wall, but when it's you at fifty-two, it's not so funny. after quite a few doctor visits, an MRI was ordered which revealed something. So they ordered a second MRI, this time with contrast. The second MRI revealed a pituitary macroadenoma, a tumor though they said that most are not cancer. I was scared to death. I had no mate, just God. And the treatment was "devil's pill." Ironic, right? This pill was supposed to shrink the tumor and by June 2015, a subsequent MRI showed that it looked like the medication was working. But to me, the mass looked the same as it had the month before. They said it was just scar tissue, and that I could discontinue the medication, I was healed.

Well you know by now that I'm the first to praise God, but something was a little off in my gut. Yet I did what they told me to do, they have the medical degrees, right? By September, I'm falling again, migraines are back, and after losing forty pounds I gained ten back. I had no equilibrium and I felt angry, crazy, nuts. I felt like I wanted to just jump out of my skin really. I'm very angry so I went back to the endocrinologist, the doctor who treated me with the medication. I described all my symptoms and he said we should check my prolactin level. He seemed very uninterested although he did say that if my prolactin level was mildly elevated, that would explain my level of sadness. He was so casual about it all. Of course my prolactin level came back high and the doctor sent me directions on the computer.

I have so many people praying for me, but I don't believe God healed me in such a short time and then gave it back. There are days when I question whether it is cancer, and I'm very scared I will go blind as the tumor presses on my optic nerve. I go Thursday for my eye test, the first of one every three months. No MRI has been scheduled yet. And I'm still on the first go-round of the medication, so time will tell but it can only get better.

*

CHAPTER TWO

THE DIAGNOSIS

Somehow, even in the worst of times, the tiniest fragments of good survive. It was the grip in which one held those fragments that counted.
-MELINA MARCHETTA

Following a devastating diagnosis or traumatic injury, the first questions we often ask ourselves are how am I going to survive this? How can I function? How can I cook and clean and cope? There we stand in the aftermath, feeling vulnerable and often ravaged with fear. Where do we go from here?

*

CHRISTINE BASTONE
Christine became ill with chronic
fatigue syndrome at the age of 27

I knew what I had, so it wasn't a surprise when I was diagnosed at age thirty-five. I quit my job not long after, as it became too much, but I think that was more of a coincidence than a consequence of the diagnosis. There was relief that someone, especially a doctor, finally agreed with me, although sadly I didn't get my diagnosis in writing. At the time, I just didn't think about getting any tangible proof. I regret that now. But other than some relief and validation, it didn't really change anything for me.

*

JERED DETWILER
Jered was diagnosed with a rare liver disorder,
Glycogen Storage Disease type 1a, as an infant
and hepatocellular cancer with liver tumors at age 31

The diagnoses of hepatocellular cancer was shocking. It is something you see on TV but never really think it could happen to you, until it happens to you. I tried to ignore the severity of it, and how large of an ordeal it would be. As the months went by and at the next few appointments the reports showed slight growth. The transplant doctors recommended that I not wait so long for a transplant and that really scared me.

Being on the transplant list I can't drink alcohol, which there are times I would love to right now. I try not to think about it, and push it to the back of my mind. Right now I'm just hoping the transplant happens soon so I can get it over with. The other concern I have is once the transplant happens I will be on a lot of medications.

In the long run I think of it as trading one disease for another. I'm trading one that has given me cancer for one that I'm going to have to treat and manage for the rest of my life. Depending on how you look at it, the side effects of each are equally balanced because they both can kill me. Fortunately, right now the transplant has a much smaller chance of taking my life as I have a one-hundred percent chance of dying with what I have right now.

As far as coping, I keep myself distracted by work, spending time with my girlfriend, watching movies with my family, and playing video games. I also use my cat as a calming agent.

*

BONNIE FORSHEY
Bonnie was diagnosed with hepatitis C at age 41, rheumatoid and
osteoarthritis at age 48, diabetes and systemic lupus at age 50,
and Graves' disease and MAC disease at age 60

I was extremely upset at the diagnosis, it was like being given a death sentence. I couldn't believe that I became so sick just from taking care of a patient, when I was just doing my job. Not much was known about hepatitis C at the time I was exposed to the tainted blood splash. The biggest concern was HIV at that time, and the patient was negative. He died a couple of days later, so of course I became worried about my future. I was raising two children alone and was very concerned about losing my job, my independence and my home. There was no cure for it, and the treatment was worse than the disease.

*

VICKI HECKROTH
Vicki was diagnosed with rheumatoid
arthritis and fibromyalgia at age 45

I was scared to death. I thought I was going to be crippled the rest of my life. I had just lost my seventeen-year-old son to suicide and had a granddaughter already here and twin grandsons on the way. I wondered if I would ever have the chance to play with them. I cried endless rivers of tears. I read everything I could on my diseases. Most of the side effects from the treatments sounded just as bad as the diseases. I had to wait a couple of months to be able to get into a rheumatologist and when I did, I thought my fears were confirmed. I would never be able to give myself shots and the powerful pain medications were so addictive. I did finally agree to try a biological medication called Humira as well as methotrexate. And of course morphine and oxycodone to help manage the pain. I soon found out that methotrexate made me feel like I had the flu every day but I suffered through it for almost three years. I then switched to Arava which eventually made my hair fall out. I now wear wigs. I weaned off both Arava and Humira about three months ago and now take Orencia. My hair is growing back but is causing my COPD from the nodules in my lungs to get worse to the point that I am now on oxygen at night.

*

BRENDA L. KLEINSASSER
Brenda was diagnosed with rheumatoid arthritis at age 31
and a right frontal lobe meningioma brain tumor at age 48

I was, of course, relieved that there was finally a diagnosis of my brain tumor, and that I was not crazy after all. I was also confused because, at the time, I did not fully realize that it was an actual brain tumor, as it was only referred to as a mass, lesion or meningioma. It was not invading my brain, so how could it possibly be a brain tumor? I did however run into several complications just weeks after. I went down to the laundry room with my mother and I was getting clothes out of the washer. We then walked up the stairs to my apartment and when we got there, my legs started to feel like they were going to give out. I immediately called my neurosurgeon and he stayed on the phone with me until I started to feel better. That was a wake-up call that I really had to keep taking it easy. Short walks were okay, as they would help stimulate the brain and so my neurosurgeon encouraged that. I also went back to work full time after two weeks, and that was definitely too soon. I landed in the ER and again had a CT scan. I was once again having problems walking and was actually using a cane, just like I did in the early days of my living with rheumatoid arthritis. They did a CT scan and found that nothing was wrong, no brain bleed or trauma. I was however told to take an additional week off from work.

About a month after, I saw my neurosurgeon for my first post-op visit and to have my stitches removed. He had actually tried putting staples in but they did not hold, so I ended up with stitches.

His nurse was even confused, as she had the staple remover set out on his desk. My doctor said that when he removed my stitches, it would feel like someone was pulling my hair. I asked him how they knew how many years my meningioma brain tumor had been there. All he said was that there had been studies done about the approximate time any given meningioma was growing, as they usually grow slowly. I remember thinking about it being like the rings on a tree, so they could tell the approximate age of it. I was trying to put this all into some perspective.

He then sent me down for another CT scan and this was when the reality of what had actually happened started to set in. The radiology technician was having difficulty getting the needle in my arm for the contrast dye. The tears started streaming down my face and I started to sob. She thought I was crying because of her trying to get the needle in. It did hurt, but I had finally come to the realization that I actually had gone through a real traumatic event. I had come through it, but now I had to learn to deal with the aftermath.

What I was experiencing was frontal lobe syndrome, which is a very real thing. At the time, I thought I was going crazy because there were times when I would just start crying for no reason. I was involved with an online support group and found out that I was not crazy. The location of my tumor in the right frontal lobe is actually the high functioning level of the brain, which was causing me to become angry or quick to tears. I had come through a traumatic event and when I realized that I actually had survived it, that is when the reality set in. I was now living a very different life. I thought that I would get this thing out of my head and everything would go back to normal. That was not going to be the case. I had to learn to live with my new normal.

The coping was very challenging at times. I started journaling six months after and found that it really did help me cope. I could see the words down on paper and see how far I had come. I started blogging and found that was another great coping mechanism for me. My first year was full of crying jags. I find that it still gets intense around the anniversary date of my craniotomy. I am truly a meningioma brain tumor survivor and I have the scars and emotions to prove it.

*

DEANA MARTIN
Deana was diagnosed with chronic depression and anxiety disorder at age 26, breast cancer at age 33, and posttraumatic stress disorder at age 45 after losing both children in a car accident

After the huge blow of the mental health diagnosis when I was twenty-six, I was sure if I took the recommended medication that would mean I was indeed "crazy." I even referred to it as crazy people medicine. My doctor explained to me that it was a chemical imbalance and a disease, and if I had diabetes would I take my insulin? Of course I would. This analogy helped me cognitively to understand it wasn't that I was flawed as I had believed my entire life. However, emotionally I did not believe this. The diagnosis of mental health issues that I probably had dealt with since childhood left me feeling damaged and gave me even more a reason to not fit in anywhere. I cried all the time during my initial treatment as one trauma after another was dissected from my soul. My friends teased me because of the tears, my family teased me because they felt, as I at first did, that the medication and treatment meant I was crazy. So everything pretty much pointed to the fact that I was mentally ill. I had heard stories of my great-grandmother having shock treatment and I could recognize mental illness in others around me in my family. I had learned that mental illness has a large genetic predisposition. My life became a deep dive into my psyche to find out what was wrong with me. It has remained a task of super human strength for as long as I can remember.

The diagnosis of breast cancer and the fear of the treatments and dying just made me feel even more crazy and alone. Now not only was my mind flawed, but my physical body had rebelled against me as well.

After the diagnosis of breast cancer I spent a great deal of time concerned with death and what would become of my children. But outwardly I tried to remain cheery and made light of a lot of it to help my children keep their fear at bay. We talked a lot about death and my theories around death and how even if it did happen, which it would not (I did not believe that, but it sounded good), that I would not be gone. I would come back at night and tickle their toes and I would always let them know I was there loving them. I discussed with them my silly plans for my last wishes, which we joked about all the time. They helped me pull out my hair when it began to fall out from chemo and we laughed at the whole thing.

The only people in my family that knew my true fears were my father, my earth angel stepmother Margi, and my younger sister. But just like the death of a child, there was no way for anyone to truly understand my fear. The steroids during chemo only made the fear and paranoia worse. In my mind I knew I was dying, just as when I found the lump I knew it was cancer. The mental aspects and the PTSD were very difficult. I don't remember what, if any, antidepressants I was on at the time. I know at one point it felt like we tried every kind known to the psychiatric community. Some antidepressants gave me vice-like headaches, some made me wacky, some sedated me, and some made me hallucinate. It took trial and error of so many medications to find a regime that worked.

Today five years after the death of my children and following outpatient treatment again, we are experimenting with my medication once more. This is terrifying! Because I know the side effects of some of them too well. Needless to say, I did not die of cancer in my early thirties, I am now a fifteen-year survivor. I don't know how long that will last because I am a strong believer in the fact that our emotions, sorrow, stress and other negativity cause disease in our physical body. I spend a great deal of life in a very dark place these days since my children died in 2011. I try to use the power of positive thinking, but their death rattled my beliefs in all that I once found to be useful in managing my mental health. I function for my granddaughter, I even smile for her. I pour my heart out to those who have experienced this pain in my attempts of helping to heal hearts in honor of my children and to make them proud. But there are days I know that they are not proud of me, and possibly even angry at my continued deep sorrow.

*

LAYNE MARTIN
Layne was diagnosed with
psoriatic arthritis at age 47

By the time I was diagnosed with psoriatic arthritis, several years had passed and I had been going to various doctors for small things that were actually symptoms of psoriatic arthritis. But, nobody ever put them all together. It wasn't until after I'd had a total hip replacement and the pathology report came back stating "consider an autoimmune disease" that I was referred to a rheumatologist.

It all started about twenty years prior when I was diagnosed with hip bursitis. I just assumed it was from my chosen profession as a nurse working in a hospital. The long twelve-hour shifts on my feet with rarely a break, and constant pushing and pulling patients off and on stretchers in the ER. My doctor would injected my hip with a cortisone shot and off I would go to finish my shift. The shots worked great so it became a habit of getting one every four months or so. Next was the really bad case of dandruff. I saw my doctor and she assumed it was from stress. My husband had decided to quit his job, and move the family across the state. Soon after the move, I started a new job managing a much larger ER and had just over one hundred employees to supervise. The dandruff was severe and I had been trying to camouflage it with light colored blouses. I even dyed my hair blonde hoping the flakes would blend in as they were really noticeable against my naturally brunette hair. After a couple doses of a topical cortisone lotion the dandruff cleared up. But then I was having difficulties with a couple of toes on each foot. At first I tried various shoes, once again I just assumed it was from being on my feet, walking around the hospital going from one meeting to another in my business dress shoes. I saw a podiatrist who diagnosed Morton's neuroma. He injected my toes with cortisone and the symptoms quickly subsided for a few months. Then came the low back pain, but again I chalked it up to my profession and years of being on my feet so I started seeing a chiropractor.

When I first saw the rheumatologist and he said I had psoriatic arthritis I had no idea what he was telling me. My first thought was, "Well, at least I don't have rheumatoid arthritis." Little did I know psoriatic arthritis could be just as destructive! As a nurse, I had heard of rheumatoid arthritis and a few other autoimmune diseases such as lupus, but I had never heard of psoriatic arthritis. I just assumed, because I had never heard of it, that it was no big deal. However, when the doctor said, "You have a severe case of psoriatic arthritis and I want to start you on a biological," I was stunned. The words coming out of his mouth literally were not registering. I could hear him talking and he handed me a pamphlet but I couldn't comprehend any of it! I remember his nurse coming in and giving me a tuberculosis skin test, and a starter kit with instructions on how to give myself shots of the biological medication at home. I walked out of his office thinking, "Well, surely it's not that bad! He's just being cautious!" Little did I know what the next couple of years would bring!

I guess when I'm asked how I handled the diagnosis...I didn't! I was in complete denial. I got on the internet and did my research but it just didn't sink in. I had been misdiagnosed so many times for so many years and they were all plausible. Now suddenly, this new doctor is telling me I have this awful disease that there is no known cure for and my life would likely be shortened. I just could not wrap my brain around it!

*

DENISE PURCELL
Denise was diagnosed with fibromyalgia
and degenerative disc disease at age 45

At first it didn't seem to be a big deal. I would just do the best I could as far as changing temperatures and feeling exhausted. For pain I took Advil. I didn't want to start the other ones like Lyrica. I tried Cymbalta but that made me feel worse. The last surgery I had was devastating to me. I have always been active and athletic, but now I could hardly walk. The doctors said I couldn't just push through it, and they referred me for pain management.

*

MARYELLEN ROACH
MaryEllen was diagnosed
with fibromyalgia at age 30

At the time I was diagnosed, I didn't realize the full impact this condition would have on my life. I also didn't know it would gradually get worse. So when I was diagnosed, I wasn't upset and was actually okay with it. I would probably still feel that way if my symptoms had stayed at the level they were when I was initially diagnosed.

*

STACY ROORDA
Stacy was diagnosed with
metastatic breast cancer at age 37

It was very scary at first. I remember sitting in the cubicle waiting to be called back for the ultrasound and biopsy of the tumor. I was listening to the technicians talk to each other and other patients who were waiting their turn for a mammogram or ultrasound, and I thought of our two beautiful daughters at home. Hannah was four and her little sister Zoe was almost three. I sat there thinking I just don't have time for this, there's laundry to do, dishes to wash, games and snuggles all waiting at home. I was used to having my busy kiddos around, and they were used to me being there for them. I felt helpless and realized all I could do was pray. There's a God bigger than all this and he's in control of all of it.

They finally took me back and I watched the computer screen as they moved the ultrasound wand around to find the tumor. There it was, a big black dot that was going to completely change my life forever. The tech tried to stay pretty neutral, but I could tell she knew it was cancer. The next few weeks were a whirlwind of phone calls, appointments, tests and more tests. Each time I had to leave my daughters at home, I felt that "mom" guilt that only mothers understand. With each new appointment, my girls grew increasingly frustrated that I had to leave again. I tried my best to answer their questions without giving too many details. I became a fabulous actress around them, trying to pretend everything was normal. If this wasn't enough to rock our world, there was another surprise in store for us.

It was a late Friday afternoon and I was scheduled for a PET scan early Monday morning. I went in for routine bloodwork the week before (my fear of needles was slowing fading). A few hours later my doctor called and said, "I have a questions for you. Is there any chance you could be pregnant?" I was speechless and my mind started reeling. I slowly replied, "I guess so but why are you asking?" Matt and I hadn't used birth control since I got pregnant with Hannah as my cycle was like clockwork. All we had to do was avoid the "danger zone" and it was all good. The doctor paused, "I got your labs back from last week and the pregnancy hormone HCG is slightly elevated. I need you to come in for a blood draw right now because if there's a chance you're pregnant then we can't do the scan on Monday." Now it was my turn to pause and I remember muttering, "Okay." The doctor told me which clinic to go to and next thing I know I'm sitting in the lab staring at the wall trying to wrap my head around the possibility of a third child. All I could think of was "What does this mean?" Sure enough the results came back and I was pregnant.

I remember hearing the doctor say, "You're pregnant and if you stay pregnant then you're going to have to be treated in Seattle. The Seattle Cancer Care Alliance is the only place around that has had a patient diagnosed with cancer and pregnant at the same time." He continued to give me information, and I started to visibly shake. For some reason the concept of being pregnant was harder to wrap my mind around that the cancer diagnosis. I had decided that I could totally beat the cancer, in my mind it was a royal pain in the butt but I could get through it all and put it behind me and continue on with life. Thinking about adding a third baby to an already noisy, busy household was overwhelming. There were so many questions racing through my mind. I finally said, "Lord what does this mean?" Not only was the cancer aggressive, but it was also estrogen-positive. My body was about to start producing the one fuel the cancer thrived on. At the very moment I asked that question, I got a vivid image of a four-point harness seat belt. The message was clear: It's going to be a rough road so sit down, buckle up, stay focused on me and you will be fine.

*

LAUREN VANDAL
Lauren suffered a traumatic
brain injury at age 35

Initially I wasn't even sure what my diagnosis was. I was discharged from the hospital with no information about anything so I just presumed all was well. I had assumed it was just like having a broken leg, a bit of rest and TLC and I would be back up and running in no time. I wasn't informed it would be any different. Looking back now of course I can see how this was a ridiculous assumption due to the delicate and important nature of the brain. How can you damage something like a brain and expect no consequence?

I remember being really tired but also just running headlong back into my life. I even attended a job interview two weeks after surgery! I went out at night, visited friends and tried to carry on with my usual life. I used to say to my partner, "I just need a good night's sleep," as I thought that would cure all my ills. What it meant was I was storing up a huge slap in the face later on down the line. I was heavily in a place of denial for about nine months post surgery. And then I started to feel and understand the effects of my accident. This is when the depression, grief, despair and anxiety began and I had no idea what was wrong with me. I was very frightened and alone. My diagnosis at this point became my enemy, I did not handle what had happened well at all. I'm still not fully in acceptance and, at times, still yearn for who I used to be. I try to forget that I have issues in some aspects of my health. It's a very difficult path to tread and I spent a lot of the time fighting myself.

*

DAWN WOINOVICK

Dawn was diagnosed with depression, posttraumatic stress disorder, degenerative disc disease at age 37, and a pituitary tumor at age 52

I think I handled it better this time around. Of course it was scary and I had to do things differently. Food tastes different, smell is stronger. Migraines are horrible, you have to learn yoga, meditation, anything that helps. The medicine for the migraines is actually anti-seizure medication, and I don't have seizures so that is worrisome. I take half a pill twice a week of the "devil's pill," and my body knows when the next half is due. This time the anxiety is so far off the charts it hits the stars. So just waiting and praying I level off quick. Sweats, chills, and even numb fingers and toes. And so it goes. My words slur and I know what I want to say but it won't come out right. I have to write everything down or I forget it.

*

Disability is a matter of perception.
If you can do just one thing well,
you're needed by someone.
MARTINA NAVRATILOVA

*

CHAPTER THREE

THE FAMILY

When wealth is lost, nothing is lost. When health is lost, something is lost. -BILLY GRAHAM

Loss of our health has a far reaching ripple effect that often impacts our family in unexpected ways. Some react in fear, others in support. How much do we tell them? Will they understand?

*

CHRISTINE BASTONE
Christine became ill with chronic
fatigue syndrome at the age of 27

More than one person said that after my diagnosis, I sort of gave up and gave in to my illness. I disagree, at least with the part about giving up. I didn't have much choice but to give in to my illness a good bit. This is how I have survived! Sometimes family members are supportive, and sometimes they are not. And some things they have come to accept, or at least they no longer push me to do. But I know that they don't understand.

I'm sure at least some things must seem ridiculous! I mean I can't go swimming if I don't feel reasonably well, or if I have someplace I have to be the next day. When I do go swimming it feels like all my energy drains out of my toes. And changing from my bathing suit back into my clothes feels like climbing Mount

Everest! These kind of things sound ridiculous. Sadly that does not make them any less true. I'm sure that my illness isn't easy on any of them either. This is especially true for my husband who ends up doing way more than his share of the workload. But it's disheartening when you don't receive the understanding and acceptance that we all crave.

*

JERED DETWILER
Jered was diagnosed with a rare liver disorder,
Glycogen Storage Disease type 1a, as an infant
and hepatocellular cancer with liver tumors at age 31

When I was initially diagnosed with GSD, my mom took care of me. It was like being diagnosed with diabetes but without all the shots. I had to eat specific foods, and stay away from specific foods. My parents had to be watchful when I got sick, but we were able to live with it. There were no other people in our area who had this disease so my parents really had to learn on their own how to manage a child who had GSD.

When I was diagnosed with hepatocellular cancer in the liver tumors, my parents were there to support me. We had to go to a class that told about transplant so I could make a choice about having a transplant or not. My dad was supportive and my mom was a bit fearful of the prospect of transplant.

Since the diagnosis, my mother has taken me to all of my medical appointments. There are so many things to know, and things I have to do to get ready for a transplant and she has been the one I have relied on to help me.

*

BONNIE FORSHEY
Bonnie was diagnosed with hepatitis C at age 41, rheumatoid and osteoarthritis at age 48, diabetes and systemic lupus at age 50, and Graves' disease and MAC disease at age 60

I handled it alone, as my children were all the close family that I had. They definitely didn't need any more stress in their young lives. I did call my sister and talk to her. She lived 1,500 miles away and I needed someone to share my situation with. She was also a nurse, and I could speak candidly with her. She tried to keep my hopes up and we started emailing frequently.

*

VICKI HECKROTH
Vicki was diagnosed with rheumatoid arthritis and fibromyalgia at age 45

My family was in shock at first, though relieved. I had a hysterectomy in 1990 due to endometrial cancer so they were certain I was dying, that the cancer had returned. Although this was not quite as serious, it was still life changing for us all.

*

BRENDA L. KLEINSASSER
Brenda was diagnosed with rheumatoid arthritis at age 31 and a right frontal lobe meningioma brain tumor at age 48

My mother was really one of the few people who knew of my diagnosis, as we decided just to share with my oldest sister and brother-in-law. You see, I had only four days from the time I saw the neurosurgeon until my craniotomy. We were both in shock and did not have a lot of time to prepare. My mother was my caregiver and I was going to be staying with her for at least a week after. She was very supportive throughout the whole process. She was sitting right alongside me, on the edge of my bed, when I received the news about the meningioma just one week prior to seeing the

43

neurologist and neurosurgeon. I really think my mother was as concerned about this situation as I was.

My mother has now been gone for over four years. I am glad she was there through this whole experience. She did one of the sweetest things ever, and I will never forget this as long as I live. I even start to tear up when I think about it. Before I was wheeled into surgery, my mother bent down and gently kissed me on the cheek. I knew at that moment that she really cared and obviously was concerned. My mother would hug me, but this type of outward expression was new to me. My mother was my only visitor, as I was in the ICU for the first day and a half before I was moved to another room. I was pretty sick the whole time, so really having her there and not a lot of visitors was fine by me.

My mother was very helpful in that she had prepared meals for me ahead of time, so all I had to do was put them in the microwave. I was to do no bending of any sort, even loading my dishes in the dishwasher. When my sister and brother-in-law came to visit, I finally got to go home to my apartment. They were very supportive and helped out a great deal. Months after, I found that being alone at night was becoming extremely difficult. I had been coming to stay on weekends after my father passed away from Alzheimer's disease, one year prior to having my brain tumor removed. It was becoming more frequent and I was now also staying during the week as well. I also found out that this is also normal.

Years before, my mother had encouraged me to write my feelings down on paper. When I started blogging, she could not believe that I could write so well. I had never really written anything before and it just seemed to flow (those were her words). Another thing that happened after this traumatic event is that I became creative. One thing my mother insisted upon me doing was learning how to do Sudoku puzzles. She taught me the easy ones, usually the first two levels. She was convinced that this would help keep my brain active and sharp. I did catch on and really did enjoy it. We were now both doing something that we enjoyed. Of course I was only doing the easy levels, and my mother would finish off with the harder ones. She would also go for short walks with me, as they did help to stimulate my brain, and also helped with my rheumatoid arthritis. We had some really deep conversations. I remember one in particular before undergoing my craniotomy. She was so concerned that if I were to not make it, whether I would be prepared for Heaven. I assured her that I would be. I hadn't even really thought about that. It wasn't until the next day getting ready for the surgery when I was told that I could have a seizure, a stroke or could even die, that it did finally hit me. I think maybe that is why she kissed me on the cheek. She was really concerned too, and wanted to make sure she had done everything possible as a mother, should something go wrong. She gave me rides to work and would help out around the apartment with cleaning, etc. She continued to be encouraging as far as my writing was concerned. I wrote a blog post about her and when I finished writing it she said, "I had no idea that I did all of those things." I got to honor her by reading it again in the past tense at her funeral. I could not have survived this experience without her love and support. I was truly grateful to have her beside me.

*

DEANA MARTIN
Deana was diagnosed with chronic depression and anxiety disorder at age 26, breast cancer at age 33, and posttraumatic stress disorder at age 45 after losing both children in a car accident

I have touched base on how my family has handled my mental and physical illnesses and diagnoses. For the most part, the physical health issues were disbelieved by my family or, if it was catastrophic, I was to buck up and get through it. No one was comfortable with my fear of death or my emotions around my physical challenges. The mental diagnoses were either chastised, ignored or made me more of an odd duck, which I already was to my family. I do however have to thank my father for standing by

45

me no matter what. He is a very positive soul and often changes the subject into all I have to be grateful for when I share my sadness and sorrow. I know his heart hurts too for the trauma I have experienced, and he has been scared for not only mine but the health of all of his daughters at one time or another. Both of my sisters have also experienced multiple physical illnesses, conditions, and severe accidents leaving permanent damage. My father refuses to let negativity into his world, and this is a beautiful trait. But I know from the trauma experienced in his childhood and life in general that some of the optimism is caused by deep insecurities and are his survival skills in order to be the man he believes he needs to be for his family. I used to be able to emulate him and his optimistic outlook in my late thirties and early forties, but at age forty-five when my children were killed in 2011, my beliefs were rocked to the very core. I have discovered that optimism is a part of who we are, for on the good days it is my fallback frame of mind.

My family continues to believe I am "messed up," they do not understand my extreme lack of energy. They of course are always concerned for my physical health and I know without a shadow of a doubt that when I face the next physical challenge in my life, my sister and my father will be by my side. They are both amazing in a crisis and I know they love me to my core. They don't always like me or my actions, but they love me!

I suppose you don't have to understand someone to love them, because there are many times that it has been difficult for them to understand me or what I have endured. However, I am extremely grateful that they do not understand fully because some of it you have to have gone through to understand the emotions behind it. They each have faced their own major health issues and I am sure they too have experienced the fear and depression that accompanies loss of health.

My grandfather used to say I wear my feelings on my sleeve, some of you will know what that means and others may not. My father recently said my continued issues with complicated grief was due to me being more sensitive than most. I don't think it is either of those actually. I believe it is that I don't buy into what we were taught about emotions and how they make you look weak. I have educated myself to the point that I know how imperative it is to express emotions and share our feelings. It's not as easy for the general populous of my extremely large family and some of them have found me weak, among many other descriptive definitions of who they think I am.

My younger sister and I, as all siblings, don't always agree on things or approve of one another's actions, but she told me that I am her hero for surviving breast cancer. She has not said so yet, but I believe some part of her is proud of me for surviving the worst trauma a mother can face: the loss of both my children. My sister loved my children as if they were her own, and even though in the beginning it was hard for everyone to understand, I truly believe she understands my immense pain and I believe she knows that I will grieve my children forever.

We have had our issues through life but truth be told, she is my hero for standing by me through all my health challenges, trying to understand my mental illness, and being strong enough to lead me around while burying my children. My sister is the strongest woman I know. She knows no defeat and she doesn't need a cape, it is very evident to all that she is a super hero in her own right!

*

LAYNE MARTIN
Layne was diagnosed with
psoriatic arthritis at age 47

I didn't really share much with my family and what I did share, I made light of. I guess I didn't share much partly because I was in denial myself and I didn't want to alarm anyone. My kids were just becoming young adults, finishing college and flying the nest. I didn't want them worried about dear old mom back at home. My husband at the time was a drama queen and had his own issues and garbage to deal with. If I had made a big deal about it, he would have come up with something bigger so there was really no point in sharing much with him.

As far as my parents and siblings, I just didn't know what to say. I didn't really understand the disease myself and it was difficult to explain. Most people think of arthritis as a disease for old people. And since I was only forty-seven, it just didn't make sense to them. Nobody seemed to understand the significance of psoriatic arthritis. Some would ask if I had rheumatoid arthritis and when I would say no, they would get a puzzled look. Then they would say something like, "So, you have osteoarthritis?" That would just exasperate me so I stopped trying to explain. Basically, I just didn't talk about it much.

I think the worst time was when I had a trip planned to Arizona to see my folks. The medication I was taking had significantly dropped my white count so I couldn't fight off infections. My doctor said he did not recommend I go at that particular time of year. If I did go I could easily contract Valley Fever which could be deadly with my compromised immune system. So, when I called my folks to say I had to cancel and reschedule my trip they were very disappointed, as was I. But I felt that they never really understood as my mom said, "You can wear a mask, can't you?" It made me feel like my safety was not of the utmost importance to them. Even though I knew it was, I felt awful about it and I almost felt like they didn't believe me. For weeks after I felt almost guilty, like I had let them down. I just didn't know what else to say or do to make them believe me. Then I worried what my mother had told my siblings and I wondered what they were all thinking. It was a terrible, vicious cycle of guilt, shame, anger and hurt. And it all had to do with this terrible disease that I didn't ask for and didn't fully understand. Now, I share freely with all who care to listen. But I have a much better understanding of the disease, and I have come to realize that I have to be my own best advocate. If I'm not feeling well or my lab results are not up to par, I don't mince words anymore and I'm no longer shy about telling my reasons for not coming to a family gathering. It's pretty cut and dried for me now, not murky and muddled like it was in the beginning.

*

DENISE PURCELL
Denise was diagnosed with fibromyalgia
and degenerative disc disease at age 45

They didn't say too much, they just tried to reinforce the stubborn side of me: I can't do this or do that. They really don't understand it.

*

STACY ROORDA
Stacy was diagnosed with
metastatic breast cancer at age 37

My parents were watching the girls when my cell phone rang and the doctor told me I was pregnant. I walked out of their bedroom and told them the news. My mom backed up and sat down in a chair. We all looked at each other in total disbelief and silence. Our usually noisy loud talkative family was actually silent for once. My mom asked me what it meant, and I said that I had no idea but my next visit was going to be in Seattle. I called my husband Matt at work, he paused and quietly replied, "Wow. Okay, what does that mean?" Again I had no answer. Before the pregnancy diagnosis, everyone was in agreement that it was going to really suck but we'd get through it together. Now there just were not any words except, "What does this mean??" Later on I called my mother-in-law and asked her if she was sitting down. I then said, "I need you to start praying because I'm pregnant." She asked the questions that were becoming very familiar: What does this mean for your treatment? How can you fight cancer when you're pregnant? Are there options? Is it even possible? I had no answers.

As the girls got ready for bed that night, I was holding it together long enough to not have a breakdown until after they were in bed. They had no idea yet what the new news was, and we kept most of the cancer talk for when they were not around. I kissed Hannah and said prayers with her as I admired her beautiful fiery red hair and her little pixie face. As I tucked the blankets up around her, she looked squarely at me and said, "You're a good mommy and you're going to be a mommy for a long time." My four-year-old daughter just spoke words over me that I needed to hear. I kissed her again and said, "Thank you, sweetie. You're a good daughter and you will be my daughter forever." She smiled and went to sleep. I barely made it to the bathroom before I lost it. I had so many emotions, but at that moment I was thankful. God had spoken directly to me just when I needed it.

*

LAUREN VANDAL
Lauren suffered a traumatic
brain injury at age 35

My family members were shocked but probably had a better handle on it than me due to witnessing it. They understood my need to rest better than I did. It was hard because my family live in England. They had to fly over to Ireland to visit me in the hospital and they were only ever able to visit for periods of time due to their own commitments at home. In a way I think this had made it both easier and harder for them, easier because the distance created by living in different countries allows for them to more seamlessly get on with their lives but harder because the distance is also frustrating when they want to help. My family was, I suppose just as much in the dark as I was really. The prognosis for a brain injury is so unknown that we just had to sit and wait. The advantage we had is that my brother-in-law is a general practitioner, so he was able to talk to the hospital staff and understand the terminology they were using. On the whole we were totally unprepared for what was to come and it's hard to understand the issues a brain injury can bring unless you experience it yourself.

*

DAWN WOINOVICK
Dawn was diagnosed with depression, posttraumatic stress disorder,
degenerative disc disease at age 37, and a pituitary tumor at age 52

At first my family was caring and sympathetic, but as time goes on they just use my condition as an excuse when I screw up. Sometimes they laugh at things I do, some are funny. Sometimes, though rarely, I get compassion and empathy. Others in the family have more important things going on, I have never been a priority and don't expect to become one now. With the exception of my youngest daughter Gracie, she does really try to help me. She makes me feel better, cares about me and my welfare, maybe too much. She's always there and helps anyway she can. She also brings me a lot of joy.

*

Employers have recognized for some time that it's smart business to have a diverse workforce - one in which many views are represented and everyone's talents are valued. Well, disability is part of diversity.
THOMAS PEREZ

*

CHAPTER FOUR

THE TRANSITION

A smile is the light in your window that tells others
that there is a caring, sharing person inside.
-DENIS WAITLEY

When handed a lifelong diagnosis, the one commonality we're all faced with is whether to share our health challenges with those around us. How much do we share with coworkers, neighbors and friends so they understand our condition and the life that lays ahead? Do we invite their support or their pity?

*

CHRISTINE BASTONE
Christine became ill with chronic
fatigue syndrome at the age of 27

A lot of times I try not to say anything at all. It feels like every time I so much as mention it, people look at me as if I have two heads! So most of the time I only mention it if I have no choice. Usually when I have to quit something. Most of the time when I do mention it, I don't explain a whole lot about it. I try to keep it short and sweet. I do wish that I could talk about it more. But of course I strongly dislike being looked at, or treated like, I have two heads! Although even I have grown incredibly weary of hearing myself saying things like, "I don't feel well."

*

JERED DETWILER
Jered was diagnosed with a rare liver disorder,
Glycogen Storage Disease type 1a, as an infant
and hepatocellular cancer with liver tumors at age 31

I don't get many questions about Glycogen Storage Disease or about the prospect of a transplant. Anyone who really knows about my condition is supportive. I told my bosses about the transplant and they asked to continue to be updated. There has been no real reaction good or bad, everyone who knows is pretty cool about it.

*

BONNIE FORSHEY
Bonnie was diagnosed with hepatitis C at age 41, rheumatoid and
osteoarthritis at age 48, diabetes and systemic lupus at age 50,
and Graves' disease and MAC disease at age 60

I told my coworkers, mainly because they were like a family. I was a nurse and they were all in the medical field, and helped me tremendously. They sought out information, and even covered my hours, if I had to see a doctor. They were a great source of comfort. We were all aware of the risks that were associated with nursing. I had another group of friends outside of work that I confided in. I lost quite a few of them due to fear. It is amazing how ignorant some people are. They were afraid to be around me, didn't want me to use their bathrooms or dishes.

*

VICKI HECKROTH
Vicki was diagnosed with rheumatoid
arthritis and fibromyalgia at age 45

I told the truth as best I could. I let people know that I would need more help, couldn't do as much, and would be on lifelong meds with no guarantees. My doctors told me that without the medication, I would be completely crippled within five years, and

54

with the medication I may not get any worse. I actually improved somewhat although I am completely disabled. My parents didn't understand and still don't. They act like the pain is all in my head, that I just want the pain meds. Like anyone would want to live like this or keep on fooling doctors and pretending all of these years.

*

BRENDA L. KLEINSASSER
Brenda was diagnosed with rheumatoid arthritis at age 31
and a right frontal lobe meningioma brain tumor at age 48

I did share with my boss. He said I must have been in shock, because I came in and told him like I was just going to a dentist appointment. He said I was that calm about it. I also told my supervisor at the time and a few coworkers, but not everyone. I had no problems with it being public, I was just trying to process it myself. At first after being diagnosed, I went off to a private place to have a good cry, as I was still trying to accept it. One of my coworkers asked if I was angry with her. I said no, that I was just diagnosed with a meningioma and I had to wait another week and was having a hard time dealing with it. I assured her that I was not angry with her. I just didn't fully understand what I was up against until I would see the neurologist or even get to see a neurosurgeon. There was a real possibility that this could possibly not even happen. I would not know anything for sure for another week. It was the longest week of my life.

I did continue to go to work up until September 5, 2008, just three days before the craniotomy. I didn't share with friends right away either, as my mother and I were still trying to prepare and process it. I really just got the general questions like whether I would have my hair shaved off, etc. I really didn't even know for sure. They ended just taking less than an inch off, so they could open the bone flap and get to the tumor. I just looked like I had a bad haircut and was able to cover it up. You could not even see my scars. Some were curious to see my head, and others could not stomach it. It really wasn't that bad, but I had scabs that were healing and would fall off. I remember several of my coworkers telling me that there were days that I shouldn't have been there, as I looked pretty rough. Working full time in the beginning was a big mistake and I should have known better, because I get fatigued from my rheumatoid arthritis. The worst part was dealing with the crying jags. The first year was by far the worst. Some people thought I was angry with them and trying to explain this new normal was frustrating at times, especially to friends. It was much harder to deal with than I had anticipated.

*

DEANA MARTIN

Deana was diagnosed with chronic depression and anxiety disorder at age 26, breast cancer at age 33, and posttraumatic stress disorder at age 45 after losing both children in a car accident

Most people thought I was a hypochondriac with all my health problems, both physical and mental, since I was very young. People lost respect for me because of all the health challenges I faced, often implying either that I had no immune system or I was making it up. Eye rolling was a typical response from my coworkers and management when I mentioned a new health issue or surgery I was facing.

Back in 1991, when I was diagnosed with chronic depression, mental illness was not understood at all. I was ostracized from my friends and coworkers as if it might be something contagious, or maybe I would flip out and go crazy right in front of their very eyes. Around this time is when I started learning that I could not trust anyone with information regarding my mental and physical health, for I would lose many relationships due to it. My friends and coworkers were very supportive during my battle with breast cancer, but like any trauma there were some who could not face me or my illness out of their own personal issues. I had two of my very best friends come to visit me while I was ill, one from Indiana and one from Texas, this meant the world to me.

56

Returning to work wearing a wig was hard, for everyone knew and I believe humans are self-conscious by nature. I always felt as if people were staring at me and treating me with pity. The company I worked for was very supportive, allowing me to take a week off after each chemo treatment and only work half days during my twenty-seven radiation treatments. I moved closer to work and the cancer hospital because one was close to the other and, at the time, I lived an hour from both. I don't remember people sending flowers or visiting after my surgery, but I am sure they did.

All in all people were very kind during this health crisis in my life. No one really asked questions, everyone knew what I had undergone and why, and no one seemed to be curious if I still had breasts or not. The main questions I faced were through many other health issues through life. I had one boss who told me that in Europe they do not operate on torn rotator cuffs. This indicated to me that he did not support my leave of absence to have rotator cuff surgery. I suffered over a year in severe pain due to his comment, and wanting and needing his approval.

I have had coworkers and friends question every surgery and illness I have faced. I have chronic bronchitis and sometimes I will have it four times in one year. I always have to hear comments like, "You have that again?" or "You are sick all the time." Well yes, I was and am sick very often, even more so since losing my children which has resulted in severely impacting my immune system.

Now that my mental health has become a greater challenge, I don't get a lot of questions from friends. I lost my job and twenty-five-year career due to my grief journey and sequelae, so I truly have no coworkers to ask questions.

With regards to losing my children, some people have asked me how I survive and go on. I tell them that I don't know, I just do. A great deal of the time I wish more people would ask, "How are you, how are you really?" I wish they would say, "Let's sit and talk about your life both physical and emotional, and how your life has changed since Amanda and Logan died." But they don't. No one says a word except for other bereaved parents. Even then, the conversation is more like, "Tell me about your kids. I am sure they were amazing people," for this is the language of our secret society where I now belong.

We never asked to join this society or learn the language of a broken heart or the chronically ill. Now that we are here, be it by fate, bad luck or simply a random accident, illness or event that we never believed could happen to our family, we know the questions to ask, we know what most of us desire. One sad factor of belonging to this society is most of our conversations could not and would not be accepted or understood anywhere but with each other.

*

LAYNE MARTIN
Layne was diagnosed with
psoriatic arthritis at age 47

Fortunately, I had my hip replacement surgery at the same hospital I worked at. A lot of the staff I had worked with for over twenty years so they were like family to me, and they were also my friends. When I was diagnosed with psoriatic arthritis, they had a few questions but most were very understanding and supportive. They had seen me coming to work using a cane for several months, parking in the disabled spots and even helped me get in and out of chairs at meetings. I think, in some sense, it was as much a relief for them as it was for me, as now we all knew what was wrong and why I had been in so much pain. I think the biggest concern came from my direct supervisor. She understood the dangers of me being on biologicals and coming in contact with infectious diseases. All of the managers were considered working managers so at times we were expected to work in our units. She changed my position into more of a desk job and I rarely had patient contact. My duties changed from just managing the emergency department to managing the medical-surgical unit too.

It was much easier handling questions from coworkers than it was handling questions from family and neighbors. But, I think that has to do with me being in the medical field, so there was already an understanding of autoimmune diseases and the medications used to treat it.

*

DENISE PURCELL
Denise was diagnosed with fibromyalgia
and degenerative disc disease at age 45

They would ask how I was doing, and say that things will get better. They didn't know what to say and I just left it alone.

*

STACY ROORDA
Stacy was diagnosed with
metastatic breast cancer at age 37

I was very open about what was going on because even though I'd always been a strong independent person, this was something just so big, scary and confusing. I needed to rely on everyone's prayers. By opening myself up, I got more support than I could have ever imagined. One thing that I've never been is fake: life is messy and never perfect. By opening myself up it allowed others to do the same, and it just felt right. For the most part I was positive and kept a brave front but I think that was just as much for me as anyone else.

*

LAUREN VANDAL
Lauren suffered a traumatic
brain injury at age 35

I had just moved over to Ireland so my social network was very small. The people I knew the most were at the accident anyway so they had a fairly good idea of how scary it was. I was also initially telling everyone I was fine and had no idea of the scale of what had happened. I find people tend to not know what to say, so they often say nothing aside from wishing you well. Maybe people feel intrusive asking questions, but I'd much rather be asked and have the elephant in the room addressed than people just pretending nothing's changed and misunderstanding who I am now. I am an open book and really appreciate it when people want to find out about my injury and make a real effort to understand what happened. My closest friends in England did initially send messages asking me about progress and how I was feeling and I was able to be more honest with them about the fatigue and anxiety. I started writing a blog about it very soon afterward, so everyone got to know about it through that. It made it easier for them to see my progress without feeling awkward asking.

The contact from friends has dwindled and the people in my life now work with the ebb and flow of recovery. It's been a hard lesson for everyone.

*

DAWN WOINOVICK
Dawn was diagnosed with depression, posttraumatic stress disorder, degenerative disc disease at age 37, and a pituitary tumor at age 52

Honestly, of course. Having been disabled for quite a long time now, the difference is this affects my brain, speech, walking and motor skills. As I write this, I am smiling. I have to tell people because it is inevitable that my diagnosis is going to come out. It is scary sometimes, there is actually a chance of rejection or like my family being made fun of. But we have to take a risk and put ourselves out there to live, don't we?

*

CHAPTER FIVE

SOCIAL ENGAGEMENTS

Those facing loss use a very simple calendar. Before
and after. -LYNDA CHELDELIN FELL

Social wellness is very important to our overall health, but
managing a lifelong health challenge sometimes impacts our social
calendar. How do we navigate engagements and invitations to join
others for activities our bodies can no longer handle?

*

JERED DETWILER
Jered was diagnosed with a rare liver disorder,
Glycogen Storage Disease type 1a, as an infant
and hepatocellular cancer with liver tumors at age 31

I'm not super physically active. I don't participate in sports
generally but I have no issue with regular daily activities. If I'm
invited to go do something, I can usually participate. I just have to
make sure I eat within the activity time to keep my blood sugar up.

*

BONNIE FORSHEY
Bonnie was diagnosed with hepatitis C at age 41, rheumatoid and
osteoarthritis at age 48, diabetes and systemic lupus at age 50,
and Graves' disease and MAC disease at age 60

I have been sick for so long that I no longer get invitations. I
have been in bed for the past ten years. I have extreme fatigue,
nausea, vomiting and chronic pain. The least little thing will tire me
out, so I don't do very much. I have lost my independence and
sense of well-being. In the early stages of my illness, I was always
a people-pleaser and could never say no. I was there for everyone
because I didn't want them to know how sick I was. It only made
me feel worse and also quite resentful. I had to learn to say no, and
take care of myself first. It's amazing how much better I felt when I
learned how to say no without feeling guilty.

*

VICKI HECKROTH
Vicki was diagnosed with rheumatoid
arthritis and fibromyalgia at age 45

I usually decline the invite, and have done this so many times
that others have stopped inviting me. I usually only go outside my
home for doctor appointments or my suicide survivors meeting.
Usually I make excuses such as having a headache or busy with
some other activities. When I say I don't feel well, people usually
treat me as if I am pretending when in actuality I am being totally
honest. Having an autoimmune disease is physically draining. I
have to use the spoons I am given very sparingly to make sure I
make it through the entire day.

Author's Note: For an explanation about the Spoon Theory, visit:
http://www.butyoudontlooksick.com/articles/written-by-christine/the-
spoon-theory/

*

BRENDA L. KLEINSASSER
Brenda was diagnosed with rheumatoid arthritis at age 31
and a right frontal lobe meningioma brain tumor at age 48

I am very selective of what I choose to do since having had my craniotomy. A big factor is noise. High pitched noises or people talking excessively fast or loud almost sends me to the ceiling. I really do not enjoy going out where there are large crowds. I will make an exception for a rock concert, where I can bring earplugs to wear to help drown out the noise. I have a really hard time being in a room that is crowded, as I start to get that closed in feeling and if someone happens to be too boisterous, I find that there really is no way to escape. I also have a hard time carrying on conversations. If I am not allowed to keep my train of thought, if someone interrupts, it can be gone just like that. It is truly frustrating. Another thing I find infuriating is when I am asked a question and not allowed to give the answer, because someone else jumps in. It takes me a little more time to collect my thoughts. We have a saying in the brain tumor community, "Brain surgery equals brain injury." I believe this to be true, as I feel inadequate at times and I hesitate to accept invitations to parties, etc. I can no longer attend church because of the loud noises. I had several invites after my craniotomy but I would always say, "Let me think about it." I decided in the end that I would just not be able to handle it.

I also have a hard time with shaking hands because of my other challenge, rheumatoid arthritis. Some people don't understand that a firm handshake can cause a lot of pain and suffering. I tried hiding my hands as a hint, but it never seemed to work. Also when I am hurting bad, I don't want to be touched. I also have a hard time standing for long periods of time, so I would end up sitting a lot of the time. I got tired of having to explain myself. It was just easier to not have to face it and after my craniotomy, it became apparent that I no longer could handle it.

My emotions also play another factor, in that I never know when they will hit. It can be embarrassing to start sobbing and have no explanation for it. I really am much less social since this whole experience of having had my brain tumor removed. I have accepted invitations to parties, but I remember my first one after my craniotomy. I ended up having to leave early and ended up bursting into tears when I reached the car. It was really a horrible experience. I appreciate knowing what I will be up against before accepting any kind of invitation so there are no unpleasant surprises.

*

MARLISE MAGNA
Marlise was diagnosed with epilepsy in 1996, fibromyalgia and insulin resistance in 2009, and posttraumatic stress disorder in 2014

I'm just honest and explain that if I'm able to participate I will, if not I will make the best of a bad situation. I sometimes feel sad or regretful, but it is what it is. I fully believe I will be healed in time. I mostly feel sad when I remember my times at the gym, my figure skating and epee sword fencing. I pray to return to those all soon.

*

LAYNE MARTIN
Layne was diagnosed with
psoriatic arthritis at age 47

It just depends on what the invitation is for and who it's from. If it's a family event, then as long as I'm feeling up to it I attend. However, you won't find me participating in any physical activities. I'd rather be visiting and catching up on what's new. If it's from a friend or my church group then I'll assess what kind of function it is. I used to love dancing and that's just not something I can do anymore. I learned the hard way that it's not worth getting out on the dance floor no matter how much fun everyone is having. If it's a summer event such as boating, again I have to think it through. I have two healed compression fractures in my back and going out on rough water or in a speed boat is just not a risk I'm going to take. I think the hardest part is not being able to participate in activities I used to enjoy. One of them, besides dancing, is amusement parks. A few years back I went to Disneyland and wasn't able to ride on most of the rides that I used to enjoy and looked forward to. It was very sad and I almost felt like it wasn't worth the trip or the money spent because I couldn't enjoy some of my favorite rides.

*

DENISE PURCELL
Denise was diagnosed with fibromyalgia
and degenerative disc disease at age 45

I try to avoid them, or I go and just sit there. I just get tired of explaining it to people who don't get it.

*

MARYELLEN ROACH
MaryEllen was diagnosed
with fibromyalgia at age 30

If I'm invited to an event or even just a get-together, I have to base my decision on the pain value of the activity and decide if I can handle it. I've received invitations to bowling parties, camping and hiking trips, and get-togethers that I've had to turn down because of the pain that would be encountered or because I wasn't feeling well at the time. Although it is still embarrassing to me, I am usually honest as to why I cannot attend. Sometimes I fully explain why, while other times I give a general explanation of, "I'm not feeling well and won't be able to attend."

*

STACY ROORDA
Stacy was diagnosed with
metastatic breast cancer at age 37

I sometimes decline because I know it will really wear me out that day and sometimes even for the next few days. If I do accept, then I know I'll pay for it but I'm too stubborn to give into my physical limitations.

*

LAUREN VANDAL
Lauren suffered a traumatic
brain injury at age 35

A lingering issue from my brain injury is fatigue, this is also the root of most of my frustration. Fatigue underpins everything, it affects mood, energy levels and motivation. I'm unable, at present, to attend any evening events and sometimes daytime ones too.

I don't try to hide my disability as I believe that awareness of brain injury is essential so people get told the truth. I tell them I can't come out because I'm tired, but thanks for asking. It's hard for people to understand why one day I might be able to go to the park for a walk and the next day be confined to my bed. I don't really see the point in pretending that it's anything other than what it is, I'm not ashamed of my disability and it means people get to see the real effects of this. I do sometimes get disappointed and frustrated when I can't do something but I'm coming to terms with that now. In the early days I got very upset and stressed when I couldn't attend events, a lot of that came from my expectations of myself but also other people not understanding why I wasn't "better."

To be honest, I really don't care anymore if someone thinks it's strange that I can't go somewhere, I live with this, they don't; and it's a waste of energy worrying about how others perceive me.

*

DAWN WOINOVICK

Dawn was diagnosed with depression, posttraumatic stress disorder,
degenerative disc disease at age 37, and a pituitary tumor at age 52

"Thanks for the invite, but I have limitations that don't allow
me to participate," is my response. Depending on the event there
might be something I can do like bring food, be the photographer,
or find something close by that interests me until the event is done.

*

*Writing means sharing. It's part of the human condition
to want to share things - thoughts, ideas, opinions.*
PAULO COELHO

*

CHAPTER SIX

PHYSICAL STRESS

Treasure the love you receive above all. It will survive
long after your good health has vanished.
-OG MANDINO

Physically stressful events can stretch our capacity to the limit.
Whether it is going to the grocery store, church, or a medical
appointment, what might be ordinary to others can present
extraordinary challenges for those with limited ability. How do we
manage these seemingly simple events? Do we ask for help?

*

CHRISTINE BASTONE
Christine became ill with chronic
fatigue syndrome at the age of 27

Lots and lots of emotions come up as I face getting ready to go
almost anywhere. Just going to church on Sunday morning, or even
visiting my sister from out of town at my parents' house takes so
much out of me. I get very overwhelmed. I get very irritable. I don't
want to go. I can't figure out why I said that I would go. I might
very well cry. I feel frustrated that it's so hard for me when it seems
so easy for everyone else. I feel depressed that I am able to do so
few fun things. I feel old before my time. I feel helpless to change
how I feel physically, even a little bit. I feel discouraged that I have

felt this way for so long. I worry about how I am going to make it through. I feel jealous of anyone who is energetic. I do go to church once in a while, attend a number of school events, and go to some family get-togethers. But I pay a price that is a heck of a lot more expensive than money in order to do so. And these are just the emotional costs, there are physical costs as well. And those are at least as difficult to deal with as the emotional ones.

*

JERED DETWILER
Jered was diagnosed with a rare liver disorder,
Glycogen Storage Disease type 1a, as an infant
and hepatocellular cancer with liver tumors at age 31

I'm a procrastinator. As far as moving goes, I'm still living with my parents. However there are some changes that need to take place in the home for when I do have the transplant. I need to change my room around and I can't have my cat in my room after the transplant. At times I also decline the help of others because I want things moved around my way and done to my satisfaction.

*

BONNIE FORSHEY
Bonnie was diagnosed with hepatitis C at age 41, rheumatoid and
osteoarthritis at age 48, diabetes and systemic lupus at age 50,
and Graves' disease and MAC disease at age 60

I am now fearful of everything. I no longer have my career to fall back on, and worry about my finances all of the time. I never ask for help, I am too proud for that. I just pray for a cure so I can go back to work, catch up on my bills, and have a better quality of life. I stress over everything now. I can't afford to trade my car in, and have had problems with it. I used to be able to trade it in every couple of years, now I am just trying to keep it running until I am well again. I feel such anxiety about the future, wondering if things will get better or worse. I am depressed over life in general. I worry about everything now, and that leads to flares and hospitalization.

70

*

VICKI HECKROTH
Vicki was diagnosed with rheumatoid
arthritis and fibromyalgia at age 45

Stress causes me to have anxiety attacks. I don't handle it very well at all. I don't believe I would do well at all if I had to make a major life change such as moving. I am slowly getting to where I can be in crowds of people again but even that is hard. I force myself because I do public speaking for suicide prevention but I can make myself literally sick from the anxiety building up to it.

*

BRENDA L. KLEINSASSER
Brenda was diagnosed with rheumatoid arthritis at age 31
and a right frontal lobe meningioma brain tumor at age 48

The emotion that comes up when I face a physically stressful event is the essence of feeling overwhelmed, because of not knowing if I can physically handle a challenge. If someone offers to help, of course I will accept. It is hard for me to ask for help, as in the past I have been made to feel like I was really putting some people out. I sometimes wished that I could still do all the things I used to, before being diagnosed with rheumatoid arthritis or having had a craniotomy. I get frustrated because I would like to be able to be more independent and be able to handle things without asking for help. It makes me feel angry and a bit sad too.

*

MARLISE MAGNA
Marlise was diagnosed with epilepsy in 1996, fibromyalgia and
insulin resistance in 2009, and posttraumatic stress disorder in 2014

Moments of severe anxiety! With my last move I was unable to pack at all, but I was blessed with a great moving company who helped me. The owner commented that he could see I was feeling extremely ill. I felt some embarrassment and felt old. I do accept support often when I know I simply cannot do a certain activity.

*

LAYNE MARTIN
Layne was diagnosed with
psoriatic arthritis at age 47

I actually just moved a couple of months ago to be closer to my daughter and her family. And at first, I wasn't sure it was going to happen as I couldn't afford to hire movers. My daughter and son-in-law helped by hiring movers to load the U-Haul, and my son-in-law drove it. I rode with my daughter in her car but it took three days of travel to get to our destination and my son-in-law had to go back to work. The U-Haul sat in their driveway for several days before we could get it unloaded at my new apartment. I was angry at first, not at them but at myself. I felt really helpless because I couldn't physically unload my own stuff. And, I was tired after three days of travel and just wanted to sleep in my own bed.

I found myself being curt with my family. I was frustrated, tired and overwhelmed. Besides the physical move, there was all of the other stuff that comes with relocating to a new state such as a change of address, a new bank, a new driver's license and license plates for my car. It is all overwhelming and some of them cost money, that's not easy for someone living strictly off of medical disability. It makes me feel worthless to not be able to care for myself the way a person of my age should be able to. I have always been a very strong, independent woman and I've lost a lot of my independence these past few years. I also get angry that I'm not able to afford a house and am stuck living in an apartment. I used to have nice furniture, a curio cabinet to display my beautiful things, a yard, a patio and a garden. Now I have a one-bedroom apartment that is sparsely decorated and have very few of my things from the past. A lot of it I sold just to be able to pay rent or be able to buy gifts for my family at Christmastime. This should be the peak of my life and I always figured I would still be working, and then during my retirement years I would travel. But, instead I'm living how I envisioned my life would be once I was elderly.

*

DENISE PURCELL
Denise was diagnosed with fibromyalgia
and degenerative disc disease at age 45

I've cried many times. I cry when I go to the store for groceries and come back with my feet swollen and pain in my back and legs. I cry because of the weight I put on because I can't exercise, and I know the right way to eat. So I can't find clothes that I like or that fit, and I get frustrated and won't leave the house.

*

STACY ROORDA
Stacy was diagnosed with
metastatic breast cancer at age 37

I've learned to just pace myself and know that I probably will be hurting the next day. I do feel a sense of sadness that I can't do more, but I don't dwell on it. I'm thankful for what I am capable of doing. Being thankful really helps to stay out of the victim mentality. But, having said that, it does bother me that I can't do as much as I'd like, yet I'm just grateful that I'm still here. I heard about a woman in my town who had kids in school and was confined to a wheelchair because of bone metastasize. She had to live in a nursing home temporarily until her house was modified enough for her to move around. That freaked me out but I worked through it.

*

LAUREN VANDAL
Lauren suffered a traumatic
brain injury at age 35

When big stressful events occur I either get very anxious and stressed or completely numb. Whichever reaction I have, I tend to pay for it a few days later with extreme fatigue and emotional lability (lots of crying!). The brain injury and the trauma has reset my resilience to low, so I'm unable to manage stress as well as I used to. In the early days of the injury I really had no control over anything and felt permanently stressed. This took a huge toll on my mental and physical health. I spent weeks just lying in bed feeling frightened and sad. Now I try to step back from events, take a breath and gather myself before I continue. I have come to realize that despite this accident happening there are still going to be other stresses in life and I needed to find a better way to deal with them. I meditate every day and my mindset has really changed as well, I just don't sweat the small stuff anymore. Funerals, house moves, hospital appointments and other people's illnesses are massive triggers for me as well as other people's lower emotions. If someone is angry or upset, I absorb it like a sponge. But I know now that I'm going to get triggered so I put as much self-care in place around events and factor in recovery time afterward. I accept any support offered and whilst that used to make me feel hopeless, I am grateful that I can access support when I need it.

*

DAWN WOINOVICK
Dawn was diagnosed with depression, posttraumatic stress disorder, degenerative disc disease at age 37, and a pituitary tumor at age 52

I always do more than I should, it's my nature, then I pay with really bad pain. So next time I move, I will use the fine art of giving people jobs. Angry helpers don't like helping, instead of "Let's just get it done," they drag it out. Then I cry out of pure exhaustion.

*

CHAPTER SEVEN

EMOTIONAL STRESS

Health is a state of complete physical, mental and social well-being, and not merely the absence of disease or infirmity. -WORLD HEALTH ORGANIZATION

As our anatomical and physiological systems work in tandem with our emotional well-being, when one part of our body is stressed, other parts become compromised. How do your emotions affect your physical health?

*

CHRISTINE BASTONE
Christine became ill with chronic
fatigue syndrome at the age of 27

Anger, fear, feeling upset...they all take their physical toll. I usually feel quite drained after feeling any of those emotions. But that's not the whole story. Happy and fun events, or activities, take a toll as well. Maybe not quite as much of one, but enough to make them not as happy or as fun as they should be. I do hesitate just a little in saying that my emotions have anything to do with my physical illness, just because chronic fatigue is so often considered as being all in our head. That is so not true. It is much more tied to the activities that I do, than any of my emotions. But emotions do play a limited role in my physical limitations.

*

JERED DETWILER
Jered was diagnosed with a rare liver disorder,
Glycogen Storage Disease type 1a, as an infant
and hepatocellular cancer with liver tumors at age 31

The gout in my knee flairs up at times when I have been doing heavy physical activity. However, even when I'm feeling down about the tumors and the cancer on my liver I can still go to work and get by in my everyday activities without a problem.

*

BONNIE FORSHEY
Bonnie was diagnosed with hepatitis C at age 41, rheumatoid and osteoarthritis at age 48, diabetes and systemic lupus at age 50, and Graves' disease and MAC disease at age 60

Any emotional issue causes me to have a flare-up. I have many autoimmune diseases which affect all of my major organs. Any little thing can cause a life-threatening problem for me. I have had to go on so many different medications, including antidepressants. I am constantly worrying about everything. I have started treatment for the chronic hepatitis C and, if it works, I will then start treatment for lupus and the MAC disease. My liver has to be stable in order to have those treatments. I don't know if I will even be able to have the treatment for my lungs, because the medications are so toxic to the liver. I feel like I am running inside of a hamster wheel, and getting nowhere fast.

*

VICKI HECKROTH
Vicki was diagnosed with rheumatoid
arthritis and fibromyalgia at age 45

Yes, but I force myself through them. My joints will swell up and ache, I will get migraines. Sometimes I get so bad with RA flares that I have to cancel the event or outing I was planning to attend. I will take Ambien, which is my sleeping medicine, and go to bed. I also take clonazepam for the anxiety. Sometimes it helps but more often it doesn't.

*

BRENDA L. KLEINSASSER
Brenda was diagnosed with rheumatoid arthritis at age 31
and a right frontal lobe meningioma brain tumor at age 48

When events are taking place in my life that cause stress or emotional upheaval, my rheumatoid arthritis does seem to become more active. I also deal with "barometer head" from having had my craniotomy, which is part of the head trauma or residual left behind from that experience. I find when I am going through an emotional battle, then my head will hurt as well. This is head pain, not a headache. It is a different kind of pain, like a burning sensation. It feels like my head is inflamed, just like my joints become sometimes with the rheumatoid arthritis.

I try to handle both of my challenges by finding things that are calming such as writing, which I find to be a real healing balm for me. I always tell myself, as my mother would tell me so many times, "This too shall pass." I also find that journaling during a stressful time can be very helpful as well. It helps to write out your feelings on paper. I find myself gaining a better perspective of the situation when I have had a chance to evaluate and decide what my plan of action will be for a solution.

*

MARLISE MAGNA
Marlise was diagnosed with epilepsy in 1996, fibromyalgia and
insulin resistance in 2009, and posttraumatic stress disorder in 2014

My emotions definitely have a cross effect. I only recently made the connection that stress heightens my symptoms, and then my symptoms flare my stress even more! It's a vicious cycle. I try stay calm and keep my mind busy, and use medication as needed. Prayer helps greatly also.

*

LAYNE MARTIN
Layne was diagnosed with
psoriatic arthritis at age 47

I find that I have to keep my emotions balanced or my arthritis flares. The biggest factor is keeping negativity out of my life. I have found it important to keep myself spiritually healthy as well as physically. It's very important for me to go to church every Sunday just to keep myself in balance. I love the worship part of the service and it seems to revitalize my spirit each week. I also find it much easier to deal with any negativity that might come my way.

It is also very important for me to be outside with nature on a daily basis. Whether it's a stroll at the local park or sitting on my daughter's patio listening to the birds chirping in the trees, or watching squirrels scurry about stealing the bird seed out of the feeders. It just gives me a sense of peace and keeps my anxiety at bay.

If I am having a flare then I sometimes just have to take a break from life, retreat to my apartment for a day or two and rest. Healthy living has also become a major factor in my life. Eating healthy foods, maintaining a healthy weight, and doing some form of low impact exercise daily had made a huge difference in my physical and emotional health.

*

DENISE PURCELL
Denise was diagnosed with fibromyalgia
and degenerative disc disease at age 45

Yes, anything emotional that weighs on your mind manifests in physical limitations. If I cry real hard my body feels stress and locks up. Intimate contact is also affected. I've lost mobility and a sense of self.

*

MARYELLEN ROACH
MaryEllen was diagnosed
with fibromyalgia at age 30

Emotionally stressful events play a huge roll in how I feel physically. The last job I had was extremely stressful and demanding, which accounted for my symptoms becoming worse over time. I have also been on a very difficult emotional roller coaster since losing my sister and two young nieces in a car accident in 2012. Since losing them, I left my stressful job of ten-plus years, I sold the house I purchased by myself and lived in for over nine years, and my parents sold the home we grew up in. We left the Midwest where we had lived for nearly all my life, which meant leaving all of my friends and the area I knew and we all moved to California. A month after we moved, my childhood home was bulldozed and I found one of our dogs after it had hung itself on my fence. My symptoms have become much worse in the last three years due to all of the stress and life changes. Physical pain will break down your endurance which makes everything more difficult to manage, and therefore it can be extremely difficult to handle both the physical and emotional pain at times. I have been able to survive this far with the help of God, my family, friends and my determination to not let fibromyalgia rule my life.

*

STACY ROORDA
Stacy was diagnosed with
metastatic breast cancer at age 37

I do feel more physically tired during stressful emotions, so I just try to take care of myself. I get really tired and tend to feel like I'm dragging the next day so I try to keep myself away from drama and let stuff go that I used to carry around. I've learned it just doesn't do any good to get all worked up over things.

*

LAUREN VANDAL
Lauren suffered a traumatic
brain injury at age 35

My emotions are tied into my physical self so anything emotionally taxing immediately affects my body too. Everything causes fatigue so times of high emotion, be it sadness, anxiety or even excitement can really drain my energy. I have to pace myself constantly and stick to a timetable to keep my fatigue in check. I also tend to feel pain in my surgery site when I'm stressed and get more aches and pains. Emotional stress can also cause my sensory issues to increase. I have very sensitive hearing and sight since the brain injury, and when I'm stressed I just can't handle noise or light. I have to sit somewhere very quiet and dark. I often wear earplugs and sunglasses to help reduce my sensitivity. I am getting better at coping with flares in my emotional and physical symptoms but they can be very scary. I practice mindfulness, and try to stay in the moment. I always tell myself that this too shall pass.

*

DAWN WOINOVICK
Dawn was diagnosed with depression, posttraumatic stress disorder,
degenerative disc disease at age 37, and a pituitary tumor at age 52

Yes, the more emotional it is, the more draining it is. If I head to an event, I will most definitely take a nap. If I am going to have a big day, I will go to bed earlier.

CHAPTER EIGHT

OUR SURROUNDINGS

Of all possessions, a friend is the most precious.
-HERODOTUS

With health challenges, we're sometimes faced with modifying our surroundings to accommodate our needs. This might be installing a bathtub bar or removing throw carpets to reduce the risk of falls. Seemingly simple challenges like opening a jar can suddenly become impossible. How do we cope?

*

JERED DETWILER
Jered was diagnosed with a rare liver disorder,
Glycogen Storage Disease type 1a, as an infant
and hepatocellular cancer with liver tumors at age 31

No, I don't need to move because of my loss of health. My situation is actually a little opposite. I have always lived at home because of my health condition. It is so expensive now to rent a place and to pay for living expenses that I haven't been able to afford to move out. I hope once I recover from the transplant to be able to work enough to afford my own place, possibly moving in with my girlfriend.

81

*

BONNIE FORSHEY

Bonnie was diagnosed with hepatitis C at age 41, rheumatoid and osteoarthritis at age 48, diabetes and systemic lupus at age 50, and Graves' disease and MAC disease at age 60

The loss of my health changed everything for me. I had a problem just walking and had severe pain in my joints. It was difficult to do anything. I had a hard time turning on lights, opening jars and closing buttons. I lost my energy and had devastating weakness and fatigue. I slept all of the time and even had a difficult time simply getting a bath. I had always been very independent and now I was unable to go to work or do the simplest task around the house. I had to buy attachments for my lights to be able to turn them on and off. I bought a cane to help me walk. The doctor wanted me to get a scooter, but I won't have anything to do with that. I will remain mobile as long as I can. My pain was so great that I had to have an intrathecal pain pump inserted in my spine.

*

VICKI HECKROTH

Vicki was diagnosed with rheumatoid arthritis and fibromyalgia at age 45

Yes, we had to move downstairs to a very small bedroom due to me not being able to use the stairs any longer. I have a huge five-bedroom home and the four nicest bedrooms and nicest bathroom are upstairs unused. The room I am in is so small I cannot even use my good dresser set, and it has no closet so my clothes hang in the entryway coat closet.

*

BRENDA L. KLEINSASSER
Brenda was diagnosed with rheumatoid arthritis at age 31
and a right frontal lobe meningioma brain tumor at age 48

With my rheumatoid arthritis, I purchased a stool I could sit on while doing things in the kitchen such as washing dishes, as it was just too painful to stand and my ankles would swell up so bad. After my craniotomy, I could not bend over so I had to make changes on arranging items in my apartment to be able to reach them more easily. I also have a chair in my shower as I can no longer sit in a tub, it is just too difficult with my rheumatoid arthritis to manage it. The shower chair is also very helpful because I now experience problems with motion due to having the craniotomy and if I happen to get lightheaded while in the shower, I have the chair for support.

At the beginning of my journey with rheumatoid arthritis I was using a cane and that really helped to manage stairs. My stairs are really wide so I have to walk with one foot and stop, and then walk with the other foot. It was very difficult to do at first. I did purchase a gripper to help with opening jars, as my hands are still bad some days with the rheumatoid arthritis.

Now with the aftermath of the craniotomy, looking up for something can cause instant nausea, as I also deal with benign positional vertigo at times. I can no longer tip my head back when I go to the hairdresser, so I shampoo my hair before my appointments. I also have to have my chair raised for comfort at work and home because of the rheumatoid arthritis. I got a lighter vacuum cleaner so I can still manage that chore around the apartment. I spread out my chores around the apartment and take breaks when needed. I deal with a lot of fatigue with both of these challenges.

*

MARLISE MAGNA
Marlise was diagnosed with epilepsy in 1996, fibromyalgia and
insulin resistance in 2009, and posttraumatic stress disorder in 2014

I don't have stairs in my home but I do find that walking a lot
causes an intense rise of discomfort and pain, as well as sleeping in
certain ways. The only medical equipment I make use of is a
ventilator, blood glucose monitor and blood pressure meter.

*

LAYNE MARTIN
Layne was diagnosed with
psoriatic arthritis at age 47

I've had a huge change in my living situation! Mostly because
I went through a divorce and I live alone now. There have been
times that my family has felt I should live in a house. But, there are
simple things that I just can't do like changing a light bulb or the
battery in a smoke detector. I used to be able to do those things but
my hands have been affected by the arthritis, so what used to be an
easy task is now sometimes impossible. Living in an apartment is
nice because if I need a simple task done or an appliance goes out
then I just put in a work request and the maintenance guys come
and take care of it. That also takes some financial stress away as
well. Just last week my refrigerator stopped working and within a
day it was replaced with a new one.

For a couple of years I lived in a townhouse with a small patio
and fenced-in private space. I loved the extra space but as my
arthritis has progressed and affected my knees and most recently
my Achilles tendons, the stairs were becoming difficult to
maneuver and I found the outdoor space becoming more difficult
to maintain. In fact, when I moved out the landlord charged me for
the extra weeding and sprucing up they had to do. I felt terrible
about that as I love to garden and for years I would spend hours in
my flowerbed, vegetable garden and herb gardens.

I now live in a single story, one-bedroom apartment. It's not what I pictured myself living in at the age of fifty-five! I really miss gardening and my outdoor space but I know it is just not realistic for me anymore. I've had a few bars installed in the bathroom and around the toilet area but other than that, it's easy for me to get around. I keep telling myself that at least I'm still independent and not living in an assistance living facility.

*

DENISE PURCELL
Denise was diagnosed with fibromyalgia
and degenerative disc disease at age 45

Because I couldn't exercise or walk long distances, I put on weight, which in return made it harder to walk with extra pressure. So my kids were burdened with a lot of lifting chores, like chopping wood, and mowing. They never complained, but I felt like a failure. It humbles you very fast and then becomes depression.

*

STACY ROORDA
Stacy was diagnosed with
metastatic breast cancer at age 37

So far it hasn't, but according to the doctors it will progress so my husband has already figured out where to put in an elevator. We've talked about building a house that is wheelchair friendly. While I'm thankful for that, I don't focus on the future what-ifs or when. It's too exhausting! There's so many variables that it's not worth the time to worry about it until it actually happens.

*

LAUREN VANDAL
Lauren suffered a traumatic
brain injury at age 35

The initial period after my brain injury was full of uncertainty. There was no definite prognosis as each brain injury is so individual. No one was really sure how much help I would need, or whether I needed to go back home to England. My mum was worried that I may need to go into a care home. Fortunately, I wasn't too physically or cognitively disabled so I got to go home with my partner and didn't have to adapt anything at home. I will say however that it affected me in ways I didn't expect. It made my world a lot smaller. I became bed bound at times and had a spell of agoraphobia and couldn't leave the house because I was extremely frightened about everything. So in that sense I would say my surroundings changed. I saw the same four walls an awful lot and my partner became my caregiver. This was a huge change in our living situation as I used to be so independent so we had to adjust our lifestyles significantly.

*

CHAPTER NINE

THE DARKNESS

Walking with a friend in the dark is better than
walking alone in the light. -HELEN KELLER

Dark thoughts are often not driven by a desire to end our life, rather
they are motivated by a need to end the unimaginable pain,
whether emotional or physical. Others feel an overwhelming guilt
over the idea of our disabilities burdening our family. Have you
had thoughts of suicide in the wake of your diagnosis?

*

CHRISTINE BASTONE
Christine became ill with chronic
fatigue syndrome at the age of 27

Oh gosh, yes! When life constantly takes more energy than you
have, it's very easy to think thoughts of suicide. It's not a constant
thing. And it usually doesn't last very long. There are also other
reasons that factor into my feelings. Although the biggest one,
either directly or indirectly, is my loss of health. For a long time I
pretty much just ignored such feelings. But after my sister died by
suicide in 2012, I started taking such feelings more seriously. In fact,
the first ones I had after my sister died were really scary at first. I
would go to bed and just lie there, not moving, until the feeling

went away. I felt that if I didn't let myself do anything, I couldn't hurt myself. Even though they were so short-lived, I still wanted to find a different way to deal with them. So I found two friends who I could share with when I felt that way. A lot of times what I shared with them was just something that I needed to say. It wasn't even necessarily what I believed, it was just the thoughts going around and around in my head. And getting them out of my head seemed to help.

I also read a few things that helped me. The first thing was that suicide happens when a person's pain exceeds their resources to handle that pain. And while that is simple, and being suicidal is complex, I do not find it simplistic. More than once I have taken a piece of paper, put a line down the middle of it, wrote "Reduce Pain" on one side, and "Increase Resources" on the other, and then listed ways that I could do both. Doing that exercise, even before any changes are actually made, has helped all by itself. The second thing was that when you're suicidal, you have a need for change that you would rather die than go on living without. And to use suicidal feelings as a catalyst for that change, which makes them empowering instead of so negative. I love this. And this is how I try to look at any suicidal feelings now.

So, yes. I have had thoughts of suicide as a result of my loss of health. But thankfully they have been just thoughts, and I have not been actively suicidal. And thankfully I have also found constructive ways to deal with them.

*

JERED DETWILER
Jered was diagnosed with a rare liver disorder,
Glycogen Storage Disease type 1a, as an infant
and hepatocellular cancer with liver tumors at age 31

No, I have not thought about suicide as a result of my loss of health.

*

BONNIE FORSHEY
Bonnie was diagnosed with hepatitis C at age 41, rheumatoid and
osteoarthritis at age 48, diabetes and systemic lupus at age 50,
and Graves' disease and MAC disease at age 60

I will admit that I did have suicidal ideations. My life is terrible. I put my nursing career on hold, lost my independence, my financial security and a lot of friends. I had to give up gardening, could not take care of my home, pool or myself. I began looking into Final Exit and Euthanasia groups. I didn't want to be a burden to anyone. I didn't want to lose my dignity and I didn't want to suffer. Fortunately for me, a cure is now here for chronic hepatitis C, and I am winning that battle. There are medicines to help with rheumatoid arthritis and lupus, and they can help make life tolerable. I am glad that I didn't make any hasty decisions. Life may not be easy, but it is still good.

*

VICKI HECKROTH
Vicki was diagnosed with rheumatoid
arthritis and fibromyalgia at age 45

Many times. In fact I have told my doctor that this isn't living, it is merely surviving. However because of the suicide of my son, I could never put my family through that pain again. The physical pain I feel from my diseases and the trouble I have breathing makes it hard to want to go on at times however.

*

BRENDA L. KLEINSASSER
Brenda was diagnosed with rheumatoid arthritis at age 31
and a right frontal lobe meningioma brain tumor at age 48

No, at first I wished that I didn't have to live with so much pain and it was very difficult to deal with. I cried pretty much that whole first month. I felt hopeless, but taking my life did not enter into the equation. I thought my life was over as I knew it. I was thirty-one years-old when diagnosed with rheumatoid arthritis. I had a job that I thought I might end up losing. The higher ups were pushing for me to go part-time. My rheumatologist at the time wanted me to go on disability. I was the sole breadwinner and that was not an option.

After my craniotomy I was dealing with thoughts that I might be going bonkers, because it was just too much at times, but I never thought of taking my life. I did however go through counseling to help work through my living with rheumatoid arthritis and also some other issues for coping with life in general. It was very helpful and it was only for a brief period of time. I learned that it was all right to cry and be able to share what I was going through. I have not gone through any type of counseling since my craniotomy, but I have been involved in several support groups which have helped immensely. I have those individuals who I know have my back and are a real source of encouragement. I also experience this type of support with some of my friends who live with arthritis as well.

Since my craniotomy, I can pretty much cry at the drop of a hat. I can be listening to a song, watching something on TV, or see someone else cry and that does it for me every time.

*

MARLISE MAGNA
Marlise was diagnosed with epilepsy in 1996, fibromyalgia and insulin resistance in 2009, and posttraumatic stress disorder in 2014

I have often lightly remarked that I feel like jumping off a bridge when pain levels were intolerable. That said I won't attempt suicide (again) after becoming a reborn Christian. I just would feel like it's a smack in God's face, especially after all the death situations He's pulled me out of. It's not my time to go yet and not my decision to make.

*

LAYNE MARTIN
Layne was diagnosed with
psoriatic arthritis at age 47

No. I would never do that to my family! I've had some pretty tough and challenging times and there have been days I've felt pretty crappy and wondered if I was going to survive. But suicide has never been on my radar. I can live with the pain of the arthritis! Most of my feeling crappy days have been due to the side effects from the medications they put you on to treat the arthritis. I'm to the point now that I'd rather die having lived a good happy life that I was cognitive of, rather than a crappy one where I feel terrible and can't think straight because I'm stoned or have brain fog.

*

DENISE PURCELL
Denise was diagnosed with fibromyalgia
and degenerative disc disease at age 45

No, but I've taken myself out of a lot of living activities. I can't spend a day shopping with the girls. I hate going anywhere in public because I'm embarrassed of my weight, and I feel like I've lost my old way of life. I feel like parts of me have just given up.

*

MARYELLEN ROACH
MaryEllen was diagnosed
with fibromyalgia at age 30

I have. Pain makes everything harder to handle because it can break down your endurance. During the times when the pain is overwhelming, it is extremely difficult to keep a positive attitude, especially when it lasts for longer periods of time. I wouldn't actually go through with ending my life, but during those times of extreme pain, I can understand why people who have even worse chronic pain wish for death and even kill themselves. Having those thoughts make me realize just how much the pain effects my life.

*

STACY ROORDA
Stacy was diagnosed with
metastatic breast cancer at age 37

Absolutely not, suicide takes the problems off of me and dumps it on someone else. There are days when I long to be in heaven and be done with it all, but all I have to do it look at my beautiful girls and they make me smile. With that being said, I'm certainly not judgmental about people who do have those thoughts. I've never been to the point of having absolutely no hope myself but it sounds like a very dark, lonely and sad place to be.

*

LAUREN VANDAL
Lauren suffered a traumatic
brain injury at age 35

I got very, very depressed after my accident. My depression became mixed with grief as well as mixed with anxiety, which made for a very emotionally painful time in my life. I often contemplated not existing anymore. I didn't want to cause my death by suicide, I never made any plans to do that. I just wanted to not be here anymore, to make the pain stop. I felt like I was in some parallel dimension somewhere, just locked in time and space, floating around, just existing. No one could get through that bubble I was in, I was unaware of my surroundings and the people around me; I knew they were there physically but I just couldn't connect with anything. Initially, I just got overwhelmed by these feelings and my day-to-day existence was miserable. I couldn't function and my self-care skills disappeared. I was literally too scared to even put my feet out of bed and on the floor. I lay in bed in my pajamas, not showering and not eating, wondering why this had happened to me and how unfair everything was. It felt like I had been ripped out from the inside. I have never felt so lonely and full of despair.

It was terrible because I knew there was nothing anyone could do to help me, I just had to go through it. I eventually began to meditate and read about my condition which really helped. I learned to accept my feelings and emotions as part of me, and accept that they weren't going to hurt me. So now I can just let them exist and know that they'll pass. It helped by not attaching labels to my emotions, I didn't see them as good or bad, they just "were." This decreased a lot of my self-created suffering and took some of the distress away.

*

Remember you don't need a certain number of friends,
just a number of friends you can be certain of.
AUTHOR UNKNOWN

*

CHAPTER TEN

INTIMACY

Enlightenment is the key to everything, and it is the key to intimacy, because it is the goal of true authenticity. -MARIANNE WILLIAMSON

When we have physical limitations, it sometimes impacts our ability to give and receive physical affection. Some relationships remain steady and faithful in spite of this. Others find it challenging. Has your loss of health impacted your ability to give and receive affection?

*

CHRISTINE BASTONE
Christine became ill with chronic
fatigue syndrome at the age of 27

It really doesn't affect any other relationship except for the one I have with my husband. Even hugging him is affected. Most people's hugs are short, but his, at least with me, are long. I can't stand in one place for more than a few seconds before I start looking for a place to sit down. So I have a tendency to pull away too soon. It has also affected our love life. I won't go into any details except to say that he's been very patient. Most of the time we schedule it so that I can gather my energy, but I feel very guilty about not being the wife in the bedroom that my husband needs and deserves.

*

JERED DETWILER
Jered was diagnosed with a rare liver disorder,
Glycogen Storage Disease type 1a, as an infant
and hepatocellular cancer with liver tumors at age 31

My medical condition has never hindered my ability to give and receive affection. I enjoy being with my girlfriend and hope for a long and lasting relationship.

*

BONNIE FORSHEY
Bonnie was diagnosed with hepatitis C at age 41, rheumatoid and
osteoarthritis at age 48, diabetes and systemic lupus at age 50,
and Graves' disease and MAC disease at age 60

I have a great relationship with my husband, he does so much for me, and keeps my hopes up. I do what I can, and I set goals for myself. I am still not the person that I once was, but I have adapted to my new life, and make the best out of it. I walk very slow, but at least I am still walking. I am thankful for my life, I am still here, and there might be a cure for lupus soon.

*

VICKI HECKROTH
Vicki was diagnosed with rheumatoid
arthritis and fibromyalgia at age 45

I can no longer give hugs, tightly hold or shake hands. The physical pain I feel from these types of things is unbearable. I cannot pick up or hold my grandbabies like I could with the older ones. It makes my heart break because I used to be such an affectionate person. Even my little Chihuahuas sitting on my lap can cause extensive pain at times.

*

BRENDA L. KLEINSASSER
Brenda was diagnosed with rheumatoid arthritis at age 31
and a right frontal lobe meningioma brain tumor at age 48

I have not been in a relationship with anyone while living with these two challenges. I do know that since having gone through my brain tumor experience that I possess much more empathy. I feel more deeply at times and it can really be scary to handle that much emotion.

I am not sure if I could handle a relationship, because there are so many variables to consider. Not only do I live with a debilitating chronic illness, but I also now have to deal with a lot of emotions, and some days it is even hard for me to be with myself at times. How could I possibly expect or would want to put someone else through that? It would have to be somebody who was tolerant and knew what they would be facing. Of course nothing in life is certain, but this would definitely be a tough road to travel, living with someone who deals with chronic issues lifelong. I have been quite shy when it comes to seeking out affection, as the fear of rejection is a great fear of mine. I feel out of place in many social settings, so that would be very difficult for me to do.

*

MARLISE MAGNA
Marlise was diagnosed with epilepsy in 1996, fibromyalgia and
insulin resistance in 2009, and posttraumatic stress disorder in 2014

My first husband was very supportive and understanding. My second husband simply didn't want to try and understand or even learn about my illness. My last relationship also ended because he couldn't understand me always feeling poorly. My current boyfriend is SUPER understanding and supportive. I am so blessed. It does hinder affection sometimes. When I'm sore, even touching my skin hurts, and believe me I'm a cuddle bunny, so this is a stressor.

*

LAYNE MARTIN
Layne was diagnosed with
psoriatic arthritis at age 47

I actually feel more affection toward others now than I did prior to the loss of my health. Maybe it's because you're forced to look at your own mortality and you treasure each moment you have with friends and loved ones. Also, in more recent years I've experienced more tragedy and sorrow in life. So I suppose that gives one a greater sense of appreciation, love and understanding.

Just prior to my retirement from my nursing career my youngest sister was diagnosed with stage II breast cancer that quickly spread into her bones and soon advanced to a stage IV cancer. During this time that she was fighting for her life, she was also fighting for the life of her unborn baby! That was the first really trying time that my family had ever had. It was a very scary time and we were all in shock that something like this could be happening to our family. Soon after I had to face going into early retirement I was very lonely and missed all of my coworkers and friends terribly. My family was several hours away and everyone was so consumed with my younger sister and her young family that I just never reached out to any of them.

Then, just two months later, the unthinkable happened and one of my young nieces was killed in a car accident. It was a very terrible time! None of us knew what to say or do! I remember just trying to keep busy and I kind of took charge of my sister's kitchen, putting food out for all of the family and friends as they arrived with condolences. I really didn't know what else to do. It's all pretty much a fog now but in the past we were not an openly affectionate family, now we are more open with our affections to one another.

I've often wondered if my arthritis didn't have an effect on why my husband stepped outside the boundaries of marriage. About a year prior to my retirement I developed a couple of spontaneous compression fractures in my spine from long-term steroid use. Naturally, they were painful and intimate relations was the furthest thing from my mind. My husband was a very large man, well over three hundred pounds, and I remember alluding to the fact that I wondered if I had gotten the fractures during the act of sex. I'm sure that was very hurtful to him and at the time it was my way of saying "hands off!" Now that I'm divorced and living alone I wish I had a companion. It's hard living alone and sometimes I don't sleep well because I might hear a noise outside that's unfamiliar and I worry how I would defend myself if someone were to break in.

I'm not necessarily interested in a sexual companion but just someone to share some memories with, go to the movies with, or sit and talk into the night. I'm not interested in online dating sites as I guess I'm just too old-fashioned and would rather meet someone in person. I don't go to bars or any of the local hangouts, in fact I'm not sure where those would be. I really haven't put myself out there to date and I do have concerns about whether or not anyone would even be interested in someone with my health issues. That brings up the question of when do you tell someone you have a chronic health issue? When you first start dating or do you wait until it starts to become more serious? I just don't know the answer and suppose I'll just cross that bridge if it ever happens.

Physically, I love hugs! Handshakes I shy away from for two reasons. First, my hands are often swollen and inflamed, so handshakes can be painful! Also, I take medications called biologicals that lower my resistance to fight off infections. Hands carry a lot of germs and I need to protect myself the best I can. When being introduced to someone or greeting someone I smile and greet them in a friendly manner but don't extend my hand. If it's obvious that they are wanting a handshake then I simply say, "I have arthritis and my hands are flaring today." That's it! Just short and sweet. If it's someone I know well or they have a puzzled look then I might add, "But I'll take a hug." There is no need to explain what type of arthritis I have or what medications I take. So far, everyone has been very understanding.

*

DENISE PURCELL
Denise was diagnosed with fibromyalgia
and degenerative disc disease at age 45

Limitations mean there are very few positions I can move into when intimacy arrives. I also feel old and burdensome, so why would someone love me?

*

MARYELLEN ROACH
MaryEllen was diagnosed
with fibromyalgia at age 30

I can still give and receive affection, but some people who hug me don't realize how much pain I have and that their hugs actually hurt. Sometimes I avoid hugs from people who don't know of my illness, but if it happens anyway and hurts too much, then I will explain it to them. I have found that most people do not want to hurt me and they will hug more gently once they are made aware.

*

STACY ROORDA
Stacy was diagnosed with
metastatic breast cancer at age 37

I tend to hug my kids more and appreciate the hugs I get from people. Hugging used to be fairly awkward for me but now I really appreciate them. My husband and I seem to hug more and there it a deeper meaning to them.

*

LAUREN VANDAL
Lauren suffered a traumatic
brain injury at age 35

I lost my ability to feel much of anything, my TBI sucked everything out of me. My partner and I had to rearrange our relationship. He went from boyfriend to caregiver overnight and it's been a difficult process. I often feel sad that I'm not the kind of girlfriend I want to be and feel very bad for him.

We are very much in love and have become very strong in lots of ways because of this but I'm unable at present to physically express my love, this is because the emotion overwhelms me and makes me anxious. Also, I'm tired most of the time and need to preserve energy. I suppose this means I don't seek affection as much because I feel that I'm disappointing him. But brain injuries make you curl up into a very small ball both physically and emotionally. It makes you hold tight to everything inside because release and freedom equals fear to a traumatized brain.

I do often wonder how we will redress the balance to be more of an equal partnership. It's an ongoing process as I write this. I've got a more structured timetable now so I feel I'm putting a bit more back into the practicalities of our relationship with chores, but I hope to one day make room for romance again.

I tell myself he wouldn't be here if he didn't want to be. And there have been times I've told him to go if he needs to find someone else, because I don't want to make his life miserable. But he's stuck around and even proposed to me this year!

*

*It is health that is real wealth
and not pieces of gold and silver.*
MAHATMA GANDHI

*

CHAPTER ELEVEN

THE RELATIONS

I have found the paradox that if you love until it hurts,
there can be no more hurt, only more love.
-MOTHER TERESA

For many of us, familial relationships are the cornerstones that help us stay sane; they keep us laughing, learning, loving. We speak one another's language and often finish one another's sentences. Sometimes, however, our health challenges cause a shift in familial connections that result in a larger impact than expected. Which relations, if any, have been impacted by your health?

*

CHRISTINE BASTONE
Christine became ill with chronic
fatigue syndrome at the age of 27

The relationship impacted most severely by my loss of health is my relationship with my husband. Even though I got sick about two years before I met my husband, our relationship has still been impacted the most. When we first met, I could work thirty-five hours a week relatively easily (although I still usually worked forty). I didn't have any kids yet, and I still lived with my parents. I hadn't been through too many push/crash cycles yet, so I actually felt a lot better then than I do now. But these days hubby does almost all of the errands. He goes a lot of places alone where we should go together. He does a lot of the housework. He's the one who takes the kids to fun places. And let's just say that our love life is not all that we dreamed of, by any means. I think the worst part is that my husband doesn't understand. Oh, he tries. And thankfully he accepts, and doesn't just dismiss my limitations. He also does many things he shouldn't have to do without complaint. And best of all he doesn't push me very much. So, while my loss of health has affected all of the relationships in my life, it has affected my marriage the most.

*

JERED DETWILER
Jered was diagnosed with a rare liver disorder,
Glycogen Storage Disease type 1a, as an infant
and hepatocellular cancer with liver tumors at age 31

With the Glycogen Storage Disease, the first few years of public school were difficult because I was bullied for having a large liver and I looked fat. I would try to explain my liver disorder but young kids don't understand. They just like to make fun of kids who are different. As I grew up I had one friend who stuck with me. We are still friends today. When I entered the workforce I found people treated me better than when I was a child. It didn't matter that I have a liver disorder. Now that I've been diagnosed with liver cancer my relationships with friends are the same but some people also tell me they are thinking about me or praying for me.

*

BONNIE FORSHEY

Bonnie was diagnosed with hepatitis C at age 41, rheumatoid and osteoarthritis at age 48, diabetes and systemic lupus at age 50, and Graves' disease and MAC disease at age 60

The relationship that has been impacted the hardest has been the one between myself and my daughter. I haven't been able to be there for her due to my illness. I missed out on the birth of my grandsons and many of their milestones in life. I haven't been able to be there with her to watch the children, or even be there on holidays. We, more or less, communicate via phone or internet. I am so ill, I just can't be there for her like I used to. I am praying for a cure. I miss being an active part of their lives.

*

VICKI HECKROTH

Vicki was diagnosed with rheumatoid arthritis and fibromyalgia at age 45

First would be the relationship between myself and my husband. Because of the pain from touching or hugging we are no longer able to be intimate with each other. We still maintain a close relationship of being best friends but the romance is completely gone from our marriage. Sometimes it feels like we are more like roommates than husband and wife. Second would be that of myself and the younger grandchildren. Because I am unable to cuddle or hold them, I have to find other ways of being close with them and letting them know how very much grandma loves them. It seems so unfair at times. Even getting down on the floor to play with them is difficult for me to do. I have resorted to watching kids movies with them, reading books, and lots of kisses.

*

BRENDA L. KLEINSASSER
Brenda was diagnosed with rheumatoid arthritis at age 31
and a right frontal lobe meningioma brain tumor at age 48

I had a friend for many years who I stood by and was supportive of. When I needed support the most, they were unavailable in more ways than one. This friend didn't understand my life as a brain tumor survivor. I was going through so much when I asked them to accompany me on a trip for a weekend to meet with other brain tumor survivors. My mother was dying in a nursing home, but my primary care physician insisted that I take this trip. He said I would always regret it if I didn't. He also said that it would be therapeutic for me, as I had been my mother's caregiver and needed to get away. I had really hoped it would have turned out that way, but it ended up being a horrible experience. My rheumatoid arthritis was attacking my body something fierce. Not only was I sporting an air cast on my right foot for a torn tendon, but my shoulders decided to join in the attack and I was experiencing excruciating pain with bursitis.

We had to fly on this trip and I had not flown since before my brain surgery. I had no reason to believe that I couldn't handle it. I took something so that I would not experience nausea. As soon as we took off, my head really starting feeling strange and I got sick immediately. By the time we reached our first layover, I was in pretty bad shape. I was so disoriented and was having a problem with keeping up to get to our gate. They wanted me to go to the ER but I refused, as I had fought hard for this trip. My friend accused me of being crabby. Now I had just lost my breakfast, was sporting an air cast, dealing with pain so bad that I wanted to scream, and I don't happen to act like Pollyanna. Excuse me for putting this person out. I might add that this was an all-expense paid trip on me. My mother was originally going to go with me, but she became ill and had to go into the nursing home. I was able to get her ticket refunded as we had taken out flight insurance. Her primary care physician wrote a very convincing letter to the insurance company, so there was no problem there. My mother suggested I take this other friend, as we had done so many things together in the past and always had a great time. Not this time.

The following day we had a luncheon and shared our brain tumor journeys. Right in front of the other brain tumor survivors, my friend told the group that I had an ugly personality. She said I used to be so happy-go-lucky. She didn't understand that I struggled with that flight and all the other things I was going through. I wanted to walk out of that room. I was so angry and felt so ashamed. I got up and went to another table, as it was a meet and greet. After that experience, I am sorry to say that things have never really been the same. I tried explaining what it was like, but she just didn't get it. My mother passed away the next month, in May 2011. She did attend the funeral, but I didn't feel like I could really show my true emotions, or I would again be accused of having an ugly personality. Not on the day that we were going to honor my mother. I read a tribute to her. The one blog post that I had written for her titled, "Crafts and a Mother's Love." I rewrote it in the past tense. I kept my composure and did not shed a tear that day. I have cried more tears since than I care to remember.

The last contact with my friend was when she invited me to one of her jewelry parties. I didn't care to have any contact, so I did not RSVP. That is something that she disliked more than anything. I have not heard from her since. I felt betrayed by the fact that I was always there for her. She even called me at 4 a.m. one morning crying because of a friendship that she was having a struggle with. Now I didn't say, "You woke me up from a sound sleep." I listened, as any good friend would. I could not believe how insensitive one person who was supposed to be my friend could be. She could not accept the new me. I had lost my mother who was my best friend, and when I needed support it was not there. It still stings when I think about it.

*

MARLISE MAGNA
Marlise was diagnosed with epilepsy in 1996, fibromyalgia and
insulin resistance in 2009, and posttraumatic stress disorder in 2014

My health situation has ended a few romantic relationships
due to lack of understanding.

*

LAYNE MARTIN
Layne was diagnosed with
psoriatic arthritis at age 47

All of my relationships have been impacted! I think mostly my
friends. As the arthritis progressed I stopped going to baby
showers, bridal showers, birthday parties, etc. I was just so
exhausted and I was struggling to work and keep up with the
certifications and mandatory training that my profession required.
Something had to give and unfortunately my social life was the first
thing to go. As my disease progressed and I made the agonizing
decision to retire early, my social life collapsed completely as most
of my friends were also coworkers.

Family ties have remained the same except I rarely get to see
any of them. I moved to be closer to my daughter and her family,
so now I'm thousands of miles away from my parents and siblings.
I miss out on all of the family gatherings which I know would be
good for my soul. We always laugh and have such a great time
together. But it is what it is, and all I can do is look forward to the
next time I get to see them all. I'm very thankful for the modern
technology we have these days. I'm a regular Facebook stalker and
love looking at the pictures my family posts. It helps me to feel like
I'm a part of their life on a regular basis.

*

DENISE PURCELL
Denise was diagnosed with fibromyalgia
and degenerative disc disease at age 45

My relationship with my fiancé has been impacted the most. Physically I wasn't able to go on long motorcycle rides, I was too tired all of the time, and am just in pain in general. Intimacy has also changed and I felt guilt a lot of the time. Since then we have reconnected but there are changes that are permanent. We just have to do things differently now.

*

MARYELLEN ROACH
MaryEllen was diagnosed
with fibromyalgia at age 30

The relationship with myself has been impacted the most. I used to think there wasn't anything I couldn't do, but now I'm slowly accepting that just isn't the truth anymore and I feel guilty, disappointed and/or embarrassed with myself. I know having fibromyalgia isn't my fault and I do what I can, but at the same time I still struggle with those feelings. I hope that eventually I will be able to overcome the negative feelings and learn to further accept the limitations I have because of fibromyalgia, without letting it hold me back from doing the things I can still do.

*

STACY ROORDA
Stacy was diagnosed with
metastatic breast cancer at age 37

My relationship with my kids has deepened and I feel much more protective over them. I remember when my hair started to fall out from the chemo, it didn't really fall out, it more like came out in clumps. I knew it was going to happen but was quite shocked by how much came out at one time, I thought it would be more gradual. When I could take a handful of hair at a time I decided to ask my husband to shave it. It was just a way of having some control over the situation, and I didn't want to walk around with bald patches. I told Matt I wanted the girls involved as I didn't want them being shocked and traumatized more than they already were. We explained to the girls what we were going to do, and why. I asked Hannah, the fearless five-year-old, if she wanted to give me a haircut. She was quite excited and happily went about cutting away. Zoe didn't like it at all, as she liked my long blonde hair. She sat on my lap the whole time and quietly cried against my chest. When Hannah got tired of styling my hair, Matt used the shaver and buzzed off the rest. It actually hurt quite a bit and my scalp was quite sensitive for a while. I held my composure the best I could while trying to console Zoe. I held her for as long as she needed but she always hated seeing me bald. I had to keep my wig on or a scarf around my head or she would run out of the room until I covered my head up. Hannah didn't seem to mind and liked helping me decide which hat or scarf to wear. I couldn't stand the wig and only wore it a few times as it was really itchy.

The best thing that came out of that was that my girls thought their hair would fall out if they got pregnant. A few years later both Zoe and Hannah said they wanted to have babies but they were going to adopt because they didn't want to be bald. I probably waited longer than I should have to let them know being bald had nothing to do with being pregnant! We still laugh about that one.

*

LAUREN VANDAL
Lauren suffered a traumatic
brain injury at age 35

My injury was so sudden and severe that it seemed to frighten people away. I had quite a large circle of friends but only one of them continues to make contact with me. I lost all my social network and felt very alone. It was almost as if I was of no use anymore because I couldn't be the "giver" in our relationships anymore. In hindsight I know I spent far too much time and energy running around after my friends, making sure they were okay without any regard for myself. My relationship with my partner is very different now, we missed out on that glorious "honeymoon" period because my accident happened one month after we met. He went straight into care mode and we often feel sad about the missed opportunity to be a little more carefree and romantic. In many ways we are stronger, solid as a rock, but that doesn't mean we don't mourn the loss of having more equality in our partnership. We both hope that this is temporary and that we can get back to being a couple again but it seems like a huge hill to climb when everything has been so changed and distorted.

Mostly, the biggest loss and impact has been my relationship with myself. I got lost somewhere that night. I often feel like I don't know who I'm looking at in the mirror and have spent many days crying about my loneliness and isolation. It was and still can be heartbreaking. It's hard when the foundation of your life; your hopes, dreams and ideas get ripped away. I worry that I'll never find my groove again, never shake off the apathy or feeling of uselessness that overwhelms me at times. Not trusting your own body or the world makes you shrink both physically and mentally and I'm still too scared to stretch. Imagine getting lost in a maze permanently. That's what a brain injury feels like, I hope one day to turn a corner and bump into myself and find a way out.

*

DAWN WOINOVICK
Dawn was diagnosed with depression, posttraumatic stress disorder, degenerative disc disease at age 37, and a pituitary tumor at age 52

All of my relationships have been impacted. It's not so much how people treat me as how I treat them. When your health changes drastically, you appreciate every second and the people in your life benefit from your challenges and your truthfulness. At the same time you will dissolve a relationship that has little or no value because time is so valuable.

My advice to other disabled people would be, concentrate on things
your disability doesn't prevent you doing well,
and don't regret the things it interferes with.
STEPHEN HAWKING

*

CHAPTER TWELVE

THE FAITH

You only ever grow as a human being if you're outside
your comfort zone. -PERCY CERUTTY

Health challenges can have far reaching effects in most areas of our
life, including faith. For some, faith deepens as it becomes a safe
haven for our sorrow. For others, it can be a source of
disappointment leading to fractured beliefs. One commonality
among those facing health challenges is that faith is often altered
one way or the other. Has your faith or beliefs been affected?

*

CHRISTINE BASTONE
Christine became ill with chronic
fatigue syndrome at the age of 27

My loss of health has affected my faith. My faith had already
been quite affected by going through the process of getting a
divorce. I left my first husband about two and a half years before I
started getting sick. But my loss of health only made that worse.
Even now, to some degree, it's still being impacted. I feel like I was
created to live in this world, but not given the strength that I need
to do so. This infuriates me. It also depresses me.

It's extremely disheartening to not have what you need. It's very hard to believe that God loves you, when just getting ready to go somewhere takes half a day's supply of energy. It's even harder to believe in the possibility of your prayers for anything being answered, when so many previous prayers for very basic things seem to fall on deaf ears. So while I haven't completely lost my faith, or my hope...my faith has definitely been impacted quite severely by my loss of health.

*

JERED DETWILER
Jered was diagnosed with a rare liver disorder,
Glycogen Storage Disease type 1a, as an infant
and hepatocellular cancer with liver tumors at age 31

Yes, my loss of health has impacted how I believe. There have been times I question God for giving me Glycogen Storage Disease and at times has even made me hate Him. I seem to go back and forth between hating and not caring about Him. At other times when it comes to caring about other people I still pray to God to help them.

*

BONNIE FORSHEY
Bonnie was diagnosed with hepatitis C at age 41, rheumatoid and
osteoarthritis at age 48, diabetes and systemic lupus at age 50,
and Graves' disease and MAC disease at age 60

Yes, my faith has been impacted. I have prayed for a cure for so very long, with no answer. I think we are pretty much on our own. I have suffered for thirty-five years. I search the internet daily for new treatments and information on diseases. I think we have to be proactive in our own care, no one else is going to do it for you.

*

VICKI HECKROTH
Vicki was diagnosed with rheumatoid
arthritis and fibromyalgia at age 45

My faith is very strong, however there are times when I get angry with God for letting me suffer like this. I know he doesn't give us more than we can handle but there are many times when I truly believe he thinks I am stronger than I really am. I have prayed to God to just let me go to sleep and never wake up. I have asked my family not to keep me alive on life support should the time ever arrive. However it did happen one time. I have lung nodules from the rheumatoid arthritis and I got pneumonia. I stopped breathing on my own due and passed out cold while driving. I was intubated for four days because I could not breathe on my own, and the doctors told my husband to call the girls, that I was not going to make it. During that time, I had a near-death experience. However they did not carry out my wishes, and the doctors in Sioux Falls, South Dakota, were able to bring me back. Sometimes I get angry that my wishes were not carried out yet at other times I am glad because it is more time I have with my girls and grandkids. I will say I am no longer afraid of death. During that time I was gone I went to a very peaceful place. A place where I just felt serenity. My first thoughts upon being brought back were actually anger and disbelief. I wanted to go back to the place I had been.

*

BRENDA L. KLEINSASSER
Brenda was diagnosed with rheumatoid arthritis at age 31
and a right frontal lobe meningioma brain tumor at age 48

I have always had hope. That is the one thing that I cling to. I believe in God, but to me that is a personal thing. I was very active in the church growing up. After being diagnosed with rheumatoid arthritis, I tried to continue singing in the choir but after a few years I had to give it up. It was just too hard to stand for long periods of time. I was diagnosed in 1991, and none of the medications I tried were very successful. It was almost ten years before I started taking biologicals, so a lot of damage had been done. I tried remaining active, but it was becoming more difficult. I finally stopped going to church.

After I was diagnosed with a brain tumor and had a craniotomy, other things came into the picture. I could no longer tolerate loud noises, high pitches or be around those who talk too fast or loud. I have never returned to church. I have been invited, but it is too hard to explain to someone those reasons. My faith remains strong and that is between God and I. I do know that if I did not possess hope, I would have given up a long time ago. My mother possessed a quiet faith, but it was genuine. I actually wrote that and it was published in her funeral program. She lived by example and we had many great talks about spiritual things. As I had mentioned before, she was very concerned at the time I was going to have the craniotomy in September 2008. We had a heart-to-heart talk and I assured her that I was ready if I were not to come through the surgery. I miss the fellowship and getting together with people.

Your life truly changes when you are faced with a challenge. In my case, it is two very significant ones. I cling to hope every day. That is what sustains me.

*

MARLISE MAGNA
Marlise was diagnosed with epilepsy in 1996, fibromyalgia and insulin resistance in 2009, and posttraumatic stress disorder in 2014

Not at all. I believe it's only made it stronger. If Jesus could suffer on the cross then I can suffer a little pain. I believe it will eventually turn out to be a great healing testimony!

*

LAYNE MARTIN
Layne was diagnosed with
psoriatic arthritis at age 47

My faith has become much stronger. I know for a lot of people they would question their faith and wonder why them. I've seen a lot of different religions and their practices over the years. I've seen a husband bargain with God for his wife's health. I've seen parents begging God to let their child live. I've seen prayer chains work. I've held hands with family members as they gathered around a bed and prayed for their loved one. I've stood by as a priest delivers last rites. I've witnessed the baptism of an infant that never took his first breath. Some religions are foreign to me but I always respected the patient's wishes and would stand alongside them and their loved one as they said their final goodbyes. Often times I said nothing, I just stood in the corner ready to lend a hand or offer a chair if needed.

I guess because I'm a nurse, I know that it could be so much worse. I find my faith to be comforting and it gets me through the rough days. Tomorrow is never promised to any of us so I just pray and thank God for everything I have been blessed with. I had an incredible and meaningful career, I have amazing kids and a wonderful family. I truly feel blessed!

*

DENISE PURCELL
Denise was diagnosed with fibromyalgia
and degenerative disc disease at age 45

Not at all. I'm not one to feel bitter or sorry for myself. I don't blame. It just is.

*

MARYELLEN ROACH
MaryEllen was diagnosed
with fibromyalgia at age 30

I wouldn't say my faith has been impacted, but this illness has made me question things more than anything else that has happened in my life. My sister and two young nieces moved to heaven after a car accident in 2012, but I never questioned why. I have always understood they are now in an incredibly beautiful, happy, peaceful place and they are surrounded by pure love. Knowing that, I cannot be sad for them and I know what happened wasn't some kind of punishment for them or those of us left behind.

On the other hand, I feel tortured every day with pain, stiffness, fatigue, concentration and memory issues, anxiety, depression, sleep problems, numbness in my hands, spider veins in my legs, gum and tooth sensitivity, sensitivity to loud noise, sensory overload, mood swings and the list goes on. Although I know this is not a punishment either and that God loves me tremendously, I do ask why. Why do I have so much pain? Why can't I wake up rested? Why can't I be normal? Why me? Why is the pain not taken away even when I continuously pray about it? Why is there no cure? I still have faith and hope, but those are two things that become strained at times regarding this illness.

*

STACY ROORDA
Stacy was diagnosed with
metastatic breast cancer at age 37

It has gotten stronger for sure, God really brought me to my knees and showed me that I'm strong but he's stronger, wiser and see's the overall big picture much clearer than I do. I trusted him before but I learned to really give things up to him that I thought I should bear myself.

*

LAUREN VANDAL
Lauren suffered a traumatic
brain injury at age 35

I didn't really have a belief system before my injury and the idea I had about faith was vague and not set in concrete. Since the injury my spiritual practice has become much more open and involved and to be honest it gives me a huge source of joy. I am forever reading and researching new ways to involve myself spiritually in my own life and recovery. I am not a follower of a traditional faith-based religion, I believe they are too full of rules and fear. My spiritual practice has become nature. Mother Earth.

I use the seasons and moon phases to help me take stock of things and clear out what no longer serves me. I would say I've become very rooted in the old traditions, I respect the planet and the creatures that live on it. I have a very open heart for the beauty that surrounds us. This accident taught me not to take anything for granted and that made me want to protect and nurture the earth. I don't hand my recovery over to a deity and disempower myself, I've learnt that my healing is an inside job and that is incredibly empowering. I have gained so much strength from my loss of health that I am learning every day how capable and in charge of my own healing I am. There's nothing better for the soul than bare feet on grass and the birds chirping in the trees!

*

DAWN WOINOVICK
Dawn was diagnosed with depression, posttraumatic stress disorder,
degenerative disc disease at age 37, and a pituitary tumor at age 52

My faith is stronger than ever. In fact I have become an ordained minister, something I have longed to do, and have basically been acting as but now can do more.

Being in control of your life and having realistic expectations about
your day-to-day challenges are the keys to stress management,
which is perhaps the most important ingredient to living
a happy, healthy and rewarding life.
MARILU HENNER

*

CHAPTER THIRTEEN

OUR HARDSHIPS

We are all born with a certain degree of power. The key to success is discovering this innate power and using it daily to deal with whatever challenges come our way. -LES BROWN

Health challenges are often invisible to others, yet greatly impacts our daily lives and sometimes even our self-worth. Do we hide our physical limitations for fear of not being valued? Is our wisdom worthy in lieu of our physical contribution? What has been the hardest challenge in your journey through loss of health?

*

CHRISTINE BASTONE
Christine became ill with chronic
fatigue syndrome at the age of 27

It's a toss-up between feeling useless, and how it has impacted me financially. Although a big part of why I feel so useless is how I can't work a regular job anymore, so they're really just two different parts of the whole. In addition to the money situation, I can't give my kids fun experiences like going to the park. I also can't give my kids vacations as I, or they, would like. I can't really go for a walk. Heck most of the time I can't even go swimming! I also miss out on a lot of fun. For instance, I've only been to Legoland a few times, while my husband and kids used to go every weekend. And my parents have a pool, I could probably swim there almost any time I wanted to do so. And yet I am able to do so only occasionally. Actually more like once in a blue moon!

Thankfully I am a homebody. I actually like being at home, and I have very little trouble amusing myself. I know many people who would not handle such things well at all. I think that I do an awesome job of handling such things, if I do say so myself! But it is so very hard to feel so useless, and like I am missing out.

*

JERED DETWILER
Jered was diagnosed with a rare liver disorder,
Glycogen Storage Disease type 1a, as an infant
and hepatocellular cancer with liver tumors at age 31

When I was in school and had a large liver and looked fat, I was getting bullied. I handled it like a child and I fought back, usually making them regret calling me names. I was so angry when they called me names. After my parents took me out of public school and I was home schooled I didn't have this problem.

After I became an adult, my medical insurance was another challenge. I worked full time to get insurance but even then I was sick off and on and didn't make that much money. This caused a lot of worry when I got on the transplant list. How was I going to pay for everything? Not too long after my first appointment at the transplant clinic I asked to have my hours reduced at work. Now I qualify for state Medicaid because I don't work enough hours to qualify for the medical insurance offered by my job. This has been a huge relief. The state Medicaid will now pay for the transplant and I don't have to worry about my medical bills.

*

BONNIE FORSHEY
Bonnie was diagnosed with hepatitis C at age 41, rheumatoid and
osteoarthritis at age 48, diabetes and systemic lupus at age 50,
and Graves' disease and MAC disease at age 60

The hardest challenge for me, was the loss of my
independence. I have always took care of everything on my own
like my house, my family, finances, etc. When I became ill, I had to
give up my nursing career. I could no longer keep up with my
home, the yard or my bills. I lost my self-identity as a strong female.
I became vulnerable, lost my dignity, and was unable to provide for
myself, and my family. I feel worthless. I have been undergoing
treatment and feel my strength returning. I hope I don't relapse and
am able to lead a productive life again. It has been pure hell to be
trapped in bed for so very long, with no hope for the future in sight.

*

VICKI HECKROTH
Vicki was diagnosed with rheumatoid
arthritis and fibromyalgia at age 45

My hardest challenge has been loneliness. It is hard to find
support from people, even family, who have never been in this
position. They don't understand chronic, all-over pain and seem to
think I am faking it at times. They get tired of me always wanting
to stay home.

I get told a lot that if this weather in Iowa makes me hurt so
bad and makes it hard to breathe then my husband and I should
just pack up and leave. What they don't understand is that doing
so is easier said than done. We own our home, my husband's job is
here, our girls and grandchildren are close enough to see when we
want to. We cannot just pick up and leave everything behind that
easily. And who is to say that living where else would make it any
easier? I get into many arguments with family and friends alike
over this. I wish there was a support group in my area for those

with chronic autoimmune diseases, and also that others would take the time to educate themselves. It is hard to understand how someone can be so sick when they look so healthy.

*

BRENDA L. KLEINSASSER
Brenda was diagnosed with rheumatoid arthritis at age 31
and a right frontal lobe meningioma brain tumor at age 48

With my rheumatoid arthritis, it was how I was going to continue to live with it. This was going to be for the rest of my life. Mine was progressing very rapidly in the beginning, in May 1991, when I was finally diagnosed. I had been battling various issues years prior, which were actually precursors to this disease. It took me years to find the right medication, all the while the damage was continuing. I tried support groups in the first few months of my diagnosis but I always came home feeling worse, so I stopped going. I tried to find out as much as I could, but this was before the internet so it was mainly with books or different publications. It was years later when I connected with someone on social media who showed me that you can live successfully with rheumatoid arthritis. It's all about how you approach it.

Several months after my mother passed, I found a project to be involved with. I was so excited to be contributing and I felt validated. Once I decided to change my attitude about how I was going to live with my rheumatoid arthritis, that is when things started to change. I mean that sincerely. With my brain tumor diagnosis and after, I became creative and also something changed with my personality. I have become braver. I take risks that I would have never been able to before. I began writing and when I saw a project opportunity to be involved with, I went for it. Had that been before my brain tumor diagnosis, there would have been no way. Part of what I do and how I cope is the promise I made to my mother while she was in the nursing home. She told me to live my life and grab what I want. I promised her she would always remain in my heart. I strive to keep that promise every day by spreading awareness for both rheumatoid arthritis and brain tumors.

I guess my hardest challenge was changing my mindset, but my brain tumor experience seemed to do that all on its own. I have said this time and again, living with rheumatoid arthritis and being a brain tumor survivor have turned out to be blessings for me. The two keep intersecting, and that convinced me even more that I was destined to face these challenges. I fight every day to keep my head above water and that can be very challenging when you are facing a disease like rheumatoid arthritis. To some it looks like I make it look too easy because I choose the positive end of the spectrum. It's my coping mechanism and believe me, it's harder than you think. I also never know on any given day what my rheumatoid arthritis may bring. There are many gifts and most are not wanted, but I handle it the best way I know how.

Now on the brain tumor side of things, my biggest challenge there is trying to keep my emotions in check. For the most part, I can handle all the hurdles that it causes. There are times, like with stressful situations, that frontal lobe syndrome will come into play. That is something that I cannot control. That is a residual from the location of my brain tumor. I have to remind myself that it is not my fault. I can honestly say that I would not want to go back to being the person I was before my brain tumor experience. I possess much more empathy, which I feel is a wonderful commodity. On the other side with my rheumatoid arthritis, it would be wonderful to be able to go back to how I was before it decided to attack my body. I know that is never going to happen and I have learned to accept that fact. The best way to continue to face these challenges is to always move forward.

One thing that I have said multiple times to those who live with a chronic illness is to remember to concentrate on the things you can do, and not on the things you can't.

*

MARLISE MAGNA
Marlise was diagnosed with epilepsy in 1996, fibromyalgia and
insulin resistance in 2009, and posttraumatic stress disorder in 2014

My hardest challenge is making people believe it's not an act.
Just because you can't see it, doesn't mean it's not real. Now I just
smile and wave. I know my truth and that's what matters.

*

LAYNE MARTIN
Layne was diagnosed with
psoriatic arthritis at age 47

The most difficult part for me has been the side effects from the
medications. I've always been very sensitive to medications so I
never really took much of anything in the past. The medications
used for the type of arthritis I have are very brutal and can have
some terrible side effects. Some have made my mind so foggy that
my mother worried I was getting Alzheimer's. Unfortunately, my
arthritis has progressed despite treatment so right now I'm pretty
much out of options. The only good thing about that is that my
brain fog has lifted and I can now remember why I went into the
next room and/or the conversations I had last week.

I look back on some of the patients I took care of over the years
and now understand what they were going through. It's very
frustrating when your mind is working great but your body won't
cooperate. And, I think what's even more frustrating nowadays is
getting the medical community to understand. Doctors now just
want to hand you a prescription for a quick fix and they move onto
the next patient. They are so busy entering data into the computer
that they forget to look at their patient. I want them to actually listen
to me and address my concerns. They don't seem to be concerned
about my quality of life. I feel like they are more concerned about
quantity of life rather than the quality.

*

DENISE PURCELL
Denise was diagnosed with fibromyalgia
and degenerative disc disease at age 45

The hardest challenge has been to stop thinking I have to look perfect and be perfect. I always took care of everyone else so I didn't know how to accept help. And it's okay not to be perfect, that beauty lies from within.

*

STACY ROORDA
Stacy was diagnosed with
metastatic breast cancer at age 37

Just taking the time to do things I enjoy and not pushing myself too much, it's an ongoing challenge to take care of myself as I'm a stress eater. I also struggle with how much to share with people as I don't want them worrying about me. My standard answer is that I'm doing great even if I feel run down or tired. It's just easier most of the time to avoid more questions or that worried sound in their voice or look in their eye. I know someday I might have to share really bad news so I keep it cheerful for now.

*

LAUREN VANDAL
Lauren suffered a traumatic
brain injury at age 35

I have found every aspect of my injury challenging. The loneliness that would sweep over me at times became smothering and overpowering. The loss of "self" made my heart ache. The crippling anxiety and depression made me want to give up and just fade away. The fatigue made my eyes burn and my legs like lead. The rejection by society for not being "complete" and "healthy" is totally agonizing. The emotional lability completely wore me out. The grief left me breathless. These are things that haven't gone away and for a long time they defined me.

I was no longer a person, I was a mass of anger and sadness and hopelessness. I WAS my brain injury, it was all I could talk about and think about every day. Not having a prognosis was difficult because I didn't know what I could work toward, I didn't know if I would always be this helpless. I felt incredibly vulnerable because no one could help me, nothing could be done to change it and there was no way out. I still have these issues but they no longer define me, they are part of me but not all of me. To get to this point took time and an incredible amount of self-reflection. I looked into the abyss and instead of running away like I had been doing, it was time to walk through it. I've never been so exposed and deeply honest with myself as this injury forced me to be. It was painful and hard and messy and seemed so endless but I made it. I practiced gratitude, I meditated, I felt my feelings, I looked inside myself and I finally let go. It's a cliché, but birth is called labor for a reason. It's hard and long and that's exactly what it felt like trying to get out of the cocoon of injury. I have truly been reborn and been given another chance and I am now so grateful for that. There's a quote by Rumi that says,

"If you desire healing, let yourself fall ill. Let yourself fall ill."

I had to do just that, I had to let go and fall and know that I would be okay.

*

DAWN WOINOVICK
Dawn was diagnosed with depression, posttraumatic stress disorder, degenerative disc disease at age 37, and a pituitary tumor at age 52

The hardest challenge has been dealing with the "devil's pill" side effects, the change in smell and taste. Getting a shower and seeing a bunch of hair in the tub. It's not like cancer though, so I should be grateful. The change in my eyesight, and fear of the unknown are also hard. I also have depth perception problems as well as numbness in my hands and feet. But I can't help but feel others have it worse, so I'm okay.

CHAPTER FOURTEEN

OUR DAY

Put your heart, mind, and soul into even your smallest
acts. This is the secret of success. -SWAMI SIVANANDA

Physical challenges impact our daily routine. Some find
mornings easiest while others find evening a welcome respite.
What is the hardest time of day for you, and why?

*

CHRISTINE BASTONE
Christine became ill with chronic
fatigue syndrome at the age of 27

Mornings are the hardest time of day for me unless I don't have
to get the kids off to school, or get ready to go anywhere. And then
late afternoon, early evening is the hardest time of day because
that's when I make dinner for my family. I don't sleep very well.
But, if possible, I try to ease into my day by reading my Kindle or
playing on my tablet. Most of the time I can do those things without
difficulty. But actually getting up and doing things is a whole
different story. I always feel like I've been hit by a truck in the
morning. And I usually feel like I've hit a wall in the late afternoon.
Not that there's any time of day when I actually feel good.

*

JERED DETWILER
Jered was diagnosed with a rare liver disorder,
Glycogen Storage Disease type 1a, as an infant
and hepatocellular cancer with liver tumors at age 31

In high school I used to stay up late. And then my first jobs were working at night, graveyard shift. I haven't really been a morning person since then. So I guess morning is my most difficult time, but not because of my health really, only because of my internal time clock.

*

BONNIE FORSHEY
Bonnie was diagnosed with hepatitis C at age 41, rheumatoid and
osteoarthritis at age 48, diabetes and systemic lupus at age 50,
and Graves' disease and MAC disease at age 60

Morning is the hardest for me. I have been so sick that all of my days just run together. When I wake up in the morning, I know that it is just another day of the same. I just lay in bed, in pain, taking medications all day with nothing to look forward to. I can't go out because I am so weak and it hurts too much. The only time that I do go out is whenever I have to have labs or see a doctor. Afterward, it takes me days to recover from it.

*

VICKI HECKROTH
Vicki was diagnosed with rheumatoid
arthritis and fibromyalgia at age 45

Mornings are the worst. It is hard getting out of bed knowing that as soon as my feet hit the ground the pain is going to begin. I am usually pretty stiff and swollen at that time of the day, and the medication takes at least thirty minutes to begin to work. I also wake up with a headache every day.

My second worst time is evening. My body is so tired from being pushed all day. The restless leg syndrome gets worse then too, which is something I never experienced until after having both knees replaced in August 2014. I now am unable to stand still or sit for very long because then my legs start jumping and twitching. By the end of the day they are so worn out that they just ache.

*

BRENDA L. KLEINSASSER
Brenda was diagnosed with rheumatoid arthritis at age 31
and a right frontal lobe meningioma brain tumor at age 48

With my rheumatoid arthritis, it is usually midday when the fatigue really starts to set in. And if my body is going through attack mode, then that day could end up being difficult. I do allow myself plenty of time and get up early in case there are any surprises with my rheumatoid arthritis. I really do not know what any given day will be like until I try to tackle it. By the end of the day, it is usually more difficult because of all the activity my body has experienced and fatigue can cause that to be a lot less on some days. I am always in pain, but it is something that I have learned to deal with. I gauge what my body can handle. It is paramount that I move every day, even if it is very little at times.

With being a brain tumor survivor, without a doubt night is the worst time for me. That started occurring several months after my craniotomy. It has gotten much better over time. I spent a great deal of time at my mother's apartment, when it was too painful or difficult to be alone. When she entered the hospital and ultimately went into the nursing home, I had no choice but to mentally get myself to be able to stay alone at night. I remember a conversation that we had, about my being able to do that. She was happy that I was working on it so diligently. I sought out help on how to handle being alone at night. One of the things suggested was to schedule evening chats. Social media has really been a godsend that way. If I am having a particularly difficult evening, I can go and seek out a friend which really helps a lot. It helps me to relax also, so I can get in the frame of mind to be able to rest.

I do not sleep well, as living with rheumatoid arthritis I am usually up several times during the night. Barometer head, with the residual aftermath from my craniotomy, can also make it difficult to sleep. One of the things that was suggested was getting a cap to wear. There is no scientific logic behind this, but it seems to help constrict the blood vessels, much like using caffeine, when experiencing headaches or migraines. My neurosurgeon said, "If it helps, don't knock it." I even had several caps made so I could keep one at my mother's apartment when I would stay there on weekends. It was the design of Bugs Bunny with "What's Up Doc." It really did help with that. I find myself wearing it much less frequently at this stage.

My mornings can also be difficult if I am facing a big challenge, as I have to really think about what is entailed to tackle it. I try to have things set out the night before, such as my clothes and accessories, so I am not stressing myself out the next morning. I try to always stay a step ahead, so that my life can be as calm as possible. It is really important for me as I continue to live with chronic pain or all the other things that come along with dealing with a chronic condition. I have very little stiffness involved since I started taking my biological medication over fourteen years ago, so most of my mornings are pretty good. If I am experiencing an attack, I make sure to allow myself plenty of time. I consider myself to be a morning person. Most mornings I walk to work and that also helps to stimulate my brain and also to put me in a good frame of mind to tackle the workday. Again, my two challenges are intersecting. I still deal with difficult nights at times, but I now have coping mechanisms that I can use. Writing is a very big one. It allows me to get away from what might be causing me anxiety. I journal most days, as it helps to get my thoughts down on paper and be able to look at it later and see how far I have come on these journeys.

*

MARLISE MAGNA
Marlise was diagnosed with epilepsy in 1996, fibromyalgia and
insulin resistance in 2009, and posttraumatic stress disorder in 2014

Definitely the evenings are hardest. I never battled sleeping but since the loss and subsequent diagnosis I have become an insomniac. Sometimes I'm awake seventy-two hours on end before a few hours of fitful, nightmare filled sleep. I can't really say why although I suspect it is posttraumatic stress disorder as diagnosed paired with terrible pain. It's only gotten worse and worse sadly. The worst of the worst for me is usually between 2 a.m. and 4 a.m. They say night is always darkest before the daylight breaks and that's exactly how I experience it - a pitch black void filled with deafening silence.

*

LAYNE MARTIN
Layne was diagnosed with
psoriatic arthritis at age 47

Late afternoon and evenings are the hardest time of the day. I almost always wake up feeling fairly good. I'm always stiff but once I'm up and about then I can usually get my body moving. By late afternoon I start to fade and by evening, I'm toast! Sometimes I'm so fatigued that I can't eat dinner. The fatigue virtually makes me nauseated. Napping or resting helps a little but not enough that I can maintain any kind of social life. I think a lot of it has to do with my sleep pattern. I rarely get a good night's sleep due to pain. I get up probably five times a night just to move a bit as my body gets so sore lying in bed. I got a new bed this year but it hasn't helped. The joints just become so stiff and sore when they are immobile. It's really a vicious cycle!

*

DENISE PURCELL
Denise was diagnosed with fibromyalgia
and degenerative disc disease at age 45

Mornings are hard to move around enough to loosen up so I can walk. Nights are difficult because I am up until I am so tired I pass out. Then I can't get up at a reasonable morning hour. It frustrates me and my partner. In looking back over the years, 6 p.m. would be my time. I would do my artwork and just sit in silence in gratitude.

*

MARYELLEN ROACH
MaryEllen was diagnosed
with fibromyalgia at age 30

The pain never stops, but evenings, nights and mornings are particularly difficult. I'm usually busy in the afternoon and that sometimes helps me ignore the nagging pain, but it becomes increasingly difficult as I try to relax in the evenings. It is then that I realize just how much pain I'm actually in and how exhausted I am. Nights are hard because when I go to bed it is nearly impossible to find a comfortable spot where I can rest. I usually toss and turn most of the night and wake up several times from intense pain. Restless nights make for a not so pleasant morning. Mornings are the absolute worst time of day for me because my legs and back are incredibly stiff when I wake up and the pain is consuming. Most mornings I have to stretch before I can do anything and sometimes I have to take a hot shower to help my muscles relax. Getting dressed is usually excruciating and some days it seems like an impossible task because it's so difficult to bend. Mornings are also when I find out if my day will be a good day, and I can do most of what I want, or if it will be limited to sitting on the couch resting.

*

STACY ROORDA
Stacy was diagnosed with
metastatic breast cancer at age 37

I think mornings are hardest because I have to get up with the kids and get them out the door for school. We all really look forward to being able to sleep in on the weekend. I generally get tired in the evening and by 7 p.m. I need to sit down and call it a day. I used to do evening bible studies but now I'm just so brain dead by evening that there's just no point.

*

LAUREN VANDAL
Lauren suffered a
traumatic brain injury at age 35

The lack of consistency among brain injuries means I can't schedule in strategies for my hardest time of the day as it changes. Sometimes it's the evenings when I would feel the grip of loneliness tighten as I thought about everyone else going about their business and doing fun things like eating out. I'm always too tired after 7 p.m. to do much of anything. Sometimes it's the morning if I've had a bad night's sleep. And if I feel a long day stretch ahead of me with no purpose, I can feel more anxious in the mornings. At other times it's the afternoon when the curtain of fatigue sweeps in and renders me useless for the rest of the day. This can change on a daily basis which adds to my frustration about trying to implement routine into my week.

*

DAWN WOINOVICK
Dawn was diagnosed with depression, posttraumatic stress disorder,
degenerative disc disease at age 37, and a pituitary tumor at age 52

I find that my spiritual time in the morning makes my day go a lot smoother, even if I'm feeling a bit off. Sometimes about midday I find taking a nap or meditating helps, especially if I'm headed for a busy afternoon or late day. Eating small portions of healthy food has become a must as nausea is my friend quite often. By nighttime I'm ready to relax and end my day. As with anything, you get great days and then have days when the migraines are like Tom-Toms going off in your head. And I just found out yesterday I will be on twenty-one days of antibiotics and probiotics because I have Lyme disease from a darn tick. One, yes one tick. Oh mercy. Health can change in just one day. It's amazing and kind of funny, at least that's how I see it at this very moment.

*

CHAPTER FIFTEEN

OUR FEAR

The oldest and strongest emotion of mankind is fear, and the oldest and strongest kind of fear is fear of the unknown. -H. P. LOVECRAFT

Fear can cut you like a knife and immobilize you like a straitjacket. Fear tells us that our life will never be the same, that our misfortunes will manifest themselves again, and that we are helpless. What do we fear most? Is there a way to control our fear so it doesn't control us?

*

CHRISTINE BASTONE
Christine became ill with chronic
fatigue syndrome at the age of 27

I am most afraid of being homeless. And unfortunately, due to what my health has done to our finances, it's been a real possibility. Thankfully we've been lucky, and so far we have not lost our home. Hopefully that will continue until I can bring in enough money as a writer for us to be able to pay all of our bills.

*

JERED DETWILER
Jered was diagnosed with a rare liver disorder,
Glycogen Storage Disease type 1a, as an infant
and hepatocellular cancer with liver tumors at age 31

I am most afraid that I might not get to see my girlfriend again for two reasons. First, there is a chance I may die during the transplant. Second, after the transplant I will need a more sterile environment and be closer to the hospital than where she lives right now.

*

BONNIE FORSHEY
Bonnie was diagnosed with hepatitis C at age 41, rheumatoid and osteoarthritis at age 48, diabetes and systemic lupus at age 50, and Graves' disease and MAC disease at age 60

I am afraid of never being able to recover. I feel like a geriatric patient. I am trapped in a body that does not work. I am a shell of the independent and vibrant woman that I used to be. I don't recognize the person that stares back at me in the mirror.

*

VICKI HECKROTH
Vicki was diagnosed with rheumatoid
arthritis and fibromyalgia at age 45

I am most afraid of being wheelchair-bound again and not being able to get to my doctor appointments. I have the wheelchair and the electric chair but my home is not handicapped accessible and neither is my van, so I cannot get the chairs out of the house or loaded into my van. If for some reason my husband were to pass on before me, I would be in a world of trouble. He has been a godsend to me in so many ways.

*

BRENDA L. KLEINSASSER
Brenda was diagnosed with rheumatoid arthritis at age 31
and a right frontal lobe meningioma brain tumor at age 48

My biggest fear has always been that I will end up being alone for the rest of my life. I face a lot of things on any given day, but I ultimately want friends to be able to share good and bad times with. Living with these two challenges has caused a lot of upheaval and some of my past friends could not handle it. They did not try to get to know and understand the new me. I was always being compared to what their friend was going through with their rheumatoid arthritis. Mine is not visible for the most part. Only my hands, if you look real closely. I also don't want to push others away by constantly talking about my pain or woes. I want to go out and have fun.

With my fatigue issues and limited energy at times, I have to schedule what I can handle. That does not sit well with some and it ends up that I am not included in most activities. I also am fearful of being excluded. I have experienced it in my own family. Finding out after the fact that some of my family members had been invited to participate in an activity. Why would you even mention it? It's hard enough being alone all the time, but do you have to rub my face in it? I can only imagine that other things have taken place without my knowledge. I feel left out of the loop on many things.

As someone living with a chronic illness, one of my biggest fears is exclusion. I choose to live my life with positivity and hope. That somehow comes across as bragging to some. I am also left out of conversations and even ignored by some walking right past me, when every other person is acknowledged. It reignites that fear that I will always be alone. I try to be helpful, but sometimes it seems like my help is not needed or wanted. I have been dealing with exclusion most of my life.

Even in the chronic illness community, I am not the typical person to some. I am still on my first biological medication, when many others have been failed by theirs and have had to try multiple ones. I do not fit into their lives and therefore I am excluded. I have tried to even convey to some that ignoring and leaving me out is not cool. It doesn't seem like a big deal to some, but it does to me. It truly hurts and one of the worst feelings in life to face. Even worse than the physical pain.

*

MARLISE MAGNA
Marlise was diagnosed with epilepsy in 1996, fibromyalgia and insulin resistance in 2009, and posttraumatic stress disorder in 2014

I cannot say I fear anything (besides bugs!). I guess the only real fear I have would be another loss, especially of my parents. Lately I lie awake thinking about this. I'd be utterly lost. I don't fear my own death though. I just fear not living my life before my end.

*

LAYNE MARTIN
Layne was diagnosed with
psoriatic arthritis at age 47

The future! I have nearly run out of present treatment options. My arthritis either progresses despite the treatment, or the side effects are so bad I have to go off the medication. I don't worry so much about the pain or mobility issues. I worry more about what organ the disease is going to attack. I've already had issues with my eyes and I wonder if I will eventually go blind.

I'm concerned about maintaining my independence. I really don't want to be a burden on my family. Right now it's all about doing what I can with exercise and diet so that I can maintain my independence as long as possible.

*

DENISE PURCELL
Denise was diagnosed with fibromyalgia
and degenerative disc disease at age 45

I fear most that life will never be that way again and all the things I loved to do early in the morning will be gone. I fear spending my nights alone as others are sleeping.

*

MARYELLEN ROACH
MaryEllen was diagnosed
with fibromyalgia at age 30

My symptoms have already gotten worse than they were when I was first diagnosed. I am very concerned that the symptoms will continue to become more severe over time and I'm afraid of what that means for me. More pain and fatigue would further limit my life and further lower my quality of life. Sometimes when the pain is overwhelming, I question if I could handle it, if it were to get worse.

*

STACY ROORDA
Stacy was diagnosed with
metastatic breast cancer at age 37

I'm not afraid of dying but I'm most afraid of having a long painful drawn out death. I don't want to die that way and I really don't want my family, especially my kids and husband, to witness that. I don't want to spend my last days on high levels of painkillers and be out of it. I really pray I can stay here to raise our girls and see my grandbabies, but if I don't then I know God had a different plan for all of us.

*

LAUREN VANDAL
Lauren suffered a traumatic
brain injury at age 35

Initially I was afraid of EVERYTHING. Life suddenly became a very scary thing to experience. My main issue was loss of being able to deal with uncertainty, so most things became a threat and a worry. I had very bad health anxiety for a while and was convinced I was dying of all the possible diseases. My poor doctor was wonderfully understanding as I bounced in and out of the surgery every week. Now I'm afraid of aging with this condition and it being an unknown quantity. Will I deteriorate? Will it cause Alzheimer's? Will I be alone? I am also afraid of losing my partner and how I would cope without my rock. Loss brings up the impermanence of everything, it brings home the fact that everything ends and initially that it so hard to cope with.

I used to be pretty fearless and dive headlong into most things. My loss of health has given me a new perspective on life and whilst there are questions about the future I've learnt to stay in the present. I can't change what has happened and I don't know for sure about the future so why worry right now?

*

DAWN WOINOVICK
Dawn was diagnosed with depression, posttraumatic stress disorder,
degenerative disc disease at age 37, and a pituitary tumor at age 52

I most fear about going blind. With a pituitary tumor it can push up against your optic nerve and your sight will be gone. I have a great eye doctor who checks me every three months and covers all bases. The medicine is supposed to shrink the tumor so that's like a backup. The other fear is they say that there is no cancer, but how do they know? I'm getting a second opinion and am a bit anxious, but praying. I'm hoping that that I get a more long-term plan with more testing for a more accurate diagnosis.

CHAPTER SIXTEEN

OUR COMFORT

Life is made up, not of great sacrifices or duties, but of
little things, in which smiles and kindness, and small
obligations given habitually, are what preserve the
heart and secure comfort. -HUMPHRY DAVY

Transition sometimes feels as if we have embarked on a foreign
journey with no companion, compass, or light. Rather than fill our
bag with necessities, we often seek to fill it with emotional items
that bring us comfort. What items or rituals bring you the most
comfort?

*

CHRISTINE BASTONE
Christine became ill with chronic
fatigue syndrome at the age of 27

What comforts me most out of the things that I do for myself is
rest. Especially after I come home from being out somewhere, there
is nothing better than lying down and either reading my Kindle, or
playing a game on my tablet. What comforts me most out of the
things that other people can give me is validation and
understanding. They are in short supply. But absolutely priceless
when given.

*

JERED DETWILER
Jered was diagnosed with a rare liver disorder,
Glycogen Storage Disease type 1a, as an infant
and hepatocellular cancer with liver tumors at age 31

Not much comforts me right now so far as the transplant process goes. I just try to push things to the back of my mind and forget about my medical issues for a while.

*

BONNIE FORSHEY
Bonnie was diagnosed with hepatitis C at age 41, rheumatoid and osteoarthritis at age 48, diabetes and systemic lupus at age 50, and Graves' disease and MAC disease at age 60

The only thing that brings me comfort is the sound of my daughter and grandsons' voices. They make me want to do anything and everything possible to get well. I use whirlpools, the hot tub, and hot wax to help with the pain. My kids help me with the depression and to be able to look forward to the future.

*

VICKI HECKROTH
Vicki was diagnosed with rheumatoid arthritis and fibromyalgia at age 45

Knowing that my husband and daughters love me, believe in me, and will always be there for me. That in my most drastic times of need they and a few friends will always be there for me. Also my faith and near-death experience, knowing that death is not something to be feared but just another gateway to a new life with Jesus and those who have passed before me.

*

BRENDA L. KLEINSASSER
Brenda was diagnosed with rheumatoid arthritis at age 31
and a right frontal lobe meningioma brain tumor at age 48

Music has always been my avenue of escape. That hasn't really changed since being diagnosed with rheumatoid arthritis or being a brain tumor survivor. Writing of course is something that came into my life sometime after my craniotomy. It gives me a sense of purpose, to be able to put my thoughts on paper and have people be able to identify with that. I like to put music on while I am writing my blog posts, as it allows my creative juices to flow. I enjoy decorating my apartment. My hobby room is like an art gallery. I can look at all the photos and each one means something to me. What brings me the most comfort is being with someone who truly understands what I am going through. I can experience this through a phone conversation or having a chat face-to-face. I enjoy hanging out with my girlfriend, as we always have a great time. She puts it to me this way, "I don't always know what you are going through, but I try to understand." That means more than I can possibly say.

Going for walks and seeing nature unfold gives me great comfort. I have befriended a golden retriever, who I walk past to and from work on most days. I always look forward to seeing him. I found out a bit about him from the owner one day. I think he is lonely. He was a rescue and always wants to play. I will just stand in front of his fence and talk to him. He even allowed me to take some photos of him. He barks but when I start to talk to him he will often stop. I enjoy something as simple as a, "Good morning," greeting. It can really make my day. I enjoy listening to music on my iPod while I am walking and stimulating my brain.

*

MARLISE MAGNA
Marlise was diagnosed with epilepsy in 1996, fibromyalgia and
insulin resistance in 2009, and posttraumatic stress disorder in 2014

In the case of my illness, knowing that getting through the long
and quiet night will bring relief in the morning. Also reading my
bible and praying.

*

LAYNE MARTIN
Layne was diagnosed with
psoriatic arthritis at age 47

My family! I love being with my kids and grandkids. They
bring me great joy and give me reason to continue on. Heating
pads, long sleeved shirts and socks bring me comfort. A cup of hot
tea brings me comfort. Cuddling with my dog and a fuzzy blanket
bring me comfort. Reading a good book brings me comfort. Getting
outside and going for a leisurely walk brings me comfort. I love the
fresh air and enjoy hearing the chatter of children playing at the
park and the birds chirping in the trees.

*

DENISE PURCELL
Denise was diagnosed with fibromyalgia
and degenerative disc disease at age 45

What brings me comfort is when I have a good day and am
able to take a ride or just not be in pain. I don't get many of them
anymore.

*

STACY ROORDA
Stacy was diagnosed with
metastatic breast cancer at age 37

Prayer. I feel like my conversations with Jesus really help me sort out answers to things. I can talk with him any time I want and that is very comforting to me. I'm very honest with him so if I'm mad or upset by something, he hears about it first! I'm also quick to give thanks for all the little things. I always tell my girls, a thankful heart is a happy heart. It's so true!

*

LAUREN VANDAL
Lauren suffered a traumatic
brain injury at age 35

I find comfort in the small things, the things that are beyond materialism and acquiring stuff. I find comfort in nature, animals, my partner, writing, reading, good food, love, sunshine, meditating and my spiritual practice. I suppose this has changed over time to a much more simplistic way of being. I find joy in peace, calm and quiet where I get to sit and breathe. This brings great comfort and stability. I no longer crave the rush and buzz of what is regarded as normal living. I have slowed down and for that I'm grateful.

*

DAWN WOINOVICK
Dawn was diagnosed with depression, posttraumatic stress disorder,
degenerative disc disease at age 37, and a pituitary tumor at age 52

My faith for sure. Reading my bible, bible study, praise time. Traveling, relaxing, reading and doing yoga. Trying to keep my breathing at a steady relaxed stage, staying focused especially if I become fearful or anxious. I believe that keeping a positive attitude is crucial to healing and health for anyone dealing with health issues. And I love to snuggle with my Chihuahua, she's partially blind and I'm disabled, so she is a registered service dog. But really, we both help each other so much. Broken doesn't mean not whole.

*Love is the only law capable
of transforming grief into hope.*
LYNDA CHELDELIN FELL

*

CHAPTER SEVENTEEN

OUR SILVER LINING

Even a small star shines in darkness.
-FINNISH PROVERB

In the earliest days following loss of health, the thought that anything good can come from our experience is beyond comprehension. Yet some say there are blessings in everything, even though we might not readily recognize them. Whether one's loss reveals the kindness of a stranger or becomes the fuel to unfurl a new leaf, each silver lining, no matter how small, yields a light in the darkness. Have you discovered a silver lining in your journey?

*

CHRISTINE BASTONE
Christine became ill with chronic
fatigue syndrome at the age of 27

Unlike our society in general, I know the value of rest and renewal. I know that pushing harder isn't always the answer, and that pushing too hard can contribute to long-term problems. I know that life is a marathon, not a sprint...and that I have to pace myself. I know that illness can't always be seen. And because of that I now give everyone, including my kids, the benefit of the doubt when they say that they are sick.

*

JERED DETWILER
Jered was diagnosed with a rare liver disorder,
Glycogen Storage Disease type 1a, as an infant
and hepatocellular cancer with liver tumors at age 31

One bit of silver lining which has resulted from my loss of health was the traveling around to the Glycogen Storage Disease conferences when I was younger. I got to meet new friends and kids who had the same rare disease as me. I also got to travel around and see different parts of the country when I went to these conferences.

However the best thing that ever happened to me because I had this disorder was that I qualified for a wish through the Make-A-Wish organization. As I was unable to qualify for the military because of my health, I was granted a wish through the Make-A-Wish organization to go on an aircraft carrier that was out at sea participating in war games. I was taken on a tour and shown the entire carrier except the weapons bay, the engine room, and where the anchor is. My favorite view was from the admiral's deck. I could see the aircraft taking off and landing. I was allowed to be on deck and observe the nighttime launches. It was all very exciting. I was allowed to sit for a few minutes in an F/A-18 Hornet while the engineer went over the systems in the cockpit with me. And to this day I still have my aviation jumpsuit and patches that were given to me at that time. It was a great experience that I will never forget.

*

BONNIE FORSHEY
Bonnie was diagnosed with hepatitis C at age 41, rheumatoid and osteoarthritis at age 48, diabetes and systemic lupus at age 50, and Graves' disease and MAC disease at age 60

I have learned just how strong that I really am. I have been unable to work for ten years, and trapped in bed. I have had to cut corners and decide what I really needed and what I could live without. I have learned just how precious life is. I have become very proactive and learned to never take no for an answer. I wanted treatment and my doctor kept putting it off, telling me to wait. I emailed her, messaged her, and called her office and cell phone on a daily basis, until she finally got tired of me, and gave in. I have learned to appreciate everything in life, because we may not have a tomorrow. I used to work all of the time and never had time to enjoy life. Now that I am starting to recover, I am going to take life easy, and enjoy my daughter and grandsons.

*

VICKI HECKROTH
Vicki was diagnosed with rheumatoid
arthritis and fibromyalgia at age 45

I have become closer to my immediate family. I have learned to rely on them more and more each day. I have also learned who my true friends are, the ones who are there for me every day and try to understand my health issues instead of avoiding me. It took me a long time to see how anything good could come out of being sick like this, however with time and careful thought processing I have come to see that it is just another obstacle I need to overcome. I realize that losing my son to suicide was the worst possible event I will ever have to go through, so I am strong enough to get through this and to make something good come out of the rest of my life. Sometimes I need a little push in the right direction, but I am surviving.

*

BRENDA L. KLEINSASSER
Brenda was diagnosed with rheumatoid arthritis at age 31
and a right frontal lobe meningioma brain tumor at age 48

Since becoming a brain tumor survivor, the silver lining in all of this was definitely becoming creative. Writing is a gift that keeps on giving. I also started writing inspirational messages and even some poetry. I have made friends on social media from all over the

151

world. I have had the pleasure of sharing my story on a radio program that broadcasts all over the world. The host has become a great friend. He allowed me to read a draft of his book that he has since published. What an honor to be able to do that. There have been too many blessings to mention in regards to becoming a brain tumor survivor. I would have missed out on so much, had this experience not existed.

With regards to living with rheumatoid arthritis, that did not come as easily. I have lived with rheumatoid arthritis a lot longer than I have been a brain tumor survivor. Becoming a brain tumor survivor changed me in a lot of ways. One of the biggest changes was my attitude and how I would be able to continue to live with these challenges. That ultimately helped to change how I would face living with rheumatoid arthritis. Social media was a big part of that transformation. When I found others who were going through similar situations, I no longer felt alone. When I started taking my biological medication, my life changed in so many ways with my rheumatoid arthritis. Not only was I able to continue working full time, but my walking was getting so much better. People would comment on that. I also noticed that I had renewed strength to be able to continue this fight. I still deal with constant pain, but I can see a real difference in my outlook. I had tried so many different types of medications for almost ten years and pretty much every one failed me. I never gave up. I did a lot of research before making my final decision to try a biological medication. I get teased all of the time for my research. I like to know what I am going to be up against in any given situation. I don't do well with surprises of that nature.

I also had mentioned that I have become much more daring since my brain tumor diagnosis and craniotomy. Something took place during that procedure. I am not sure of what all that entailed, but I am definitely a different person. I strive to spread awareness every day with these two challenges. I saw an opportunity and I went for it. There is no way that would have happened had it not been for going through the trauma of having had a brain tumor removed. My battles and blessings continue to intersect. I have been able to tell my story of living with rheumatoid arthritis through a local TV and newspaper interview. I have even testified at our state capitol in North Dakota. I am now an advocate for those who feel they have no voice or are too afraid to speak up. I believe strongly in being the patient's voice. I do all of this in my mother's memory and the promise I made to her while she was dying in the nursing home. She taught me how to be a fighter, in every sense of the word.

*

MARLISE MAGNA
Marlise was diagnosed with epilepsy in 1996, fibromyalgia and insulin resistance in 2009, and posttraumatic stress disorder in 2014

I suppose the silver lining I found was to discover it's important never to take good health for granted. Every pain free moment is truly a blessing. I also found that I am able to help heal people that I lay hands on or pray for. It took me a few years to realize this and come to peace with it.

*

LAYNE MARTIN
Layne was diagnosed with
psoriatic arthritis at age 47

I think it's giving me a lot more compassion for those with chronic illnesses. And, because I'm also an R.N., it has put me at an advantage to be a patient advocate. I understand the viewpoints of the physician, hospitals, clinics, pharmaceutical companies and now the patient. I'm using that knowledge to advocate and help others with all different types of arthritis and autoimmune diseases.

*

DENISE PURCELL
Denise was diagnosed with fibromyalgia
and degenerative disc disease at age 45

It has allowed me to see that I can ask for help and get it. I don't have to be superwoman.

*

MARYELLEN ROACH
MaryEllen was diagnosed
with fibromyalgia at age 30

As a person who usually finds the good in everything, I have to say it is very difficult to find the silver lining with this illness. There are so many negative effects on me and aspects of my life that the negativity overwhelms anything positive. Digging deep to find something positive to say, I guess having this illness has helped me understand a lot of things. I now understand what others with chronic fatigue, pain, brain fog and other symptoms and conditions, go through. It has helped me be more compassionate to others and now I understand how misunderstood "invisible" illnesses are, both by the healthcare industry and society. I also recognize and appreciate the days when I feel better and can have a productive day. The main silver lining I can find is that I have the opportunity to openly talk about fibromyalgia which will hopefully help others understand and be compassionate toward those of us who have to live with this terrible illness every minute of every single day.

*

STACY ROORDA
Stacy was diagnosed with
metastatic breast cancer at age 37

I've really learned to trust God with absolutely everything. I used to be more of a self-sufficient Christian, only giving God what I thought I couldn't handle. Now I give him everything. It makes life so much easier! I've also learned to let a lot of drama go, things that used to bother me don't bother me anymore. It's given me a much better perspective on everything.

*

LAUREN VANDAL
Lauren suffered a traumatic
brain injury at age 35

At first, there was no silver lining for me. Nothing to be grateful for. Not even for being alive. What was the point of being alive if my existence was so miserable?

Slowly, slowly like the unfurling of a spring flower, I have begun to see the gifts that have come from my loss of health. It took about two years before I started to look at my injury in a more positive light and it's something that I'm still uncovering now. My brain injury has slowed me down, it has taken me out of the rush, rush, rush of everyday life. I was so firmly entrenched in "busyness" that I wasn't really living anyway. I used my job and my hobbies to cover up the deep unhappiness I felt. I never felt like I really belonged in what is considered "normal" society. I was a square peg in a round hole for much of my life. My injury has given me space to grow and breathe and realize that my happiness and my feeling of worth comes from within. Not from a job, not from how much "stuff" I own and not from wearing myself out pleasing others.

I am infinitely more patient and compassionate than I used to be, I have also learnt that there is no shame in saying no. I am also almost impossible to offend now, I'm not stuck in the minutiae of life and no longer attach my own self to the opinions of others. It has given me freedom in a way I never thought possible. I have learnt to stop and smell the roses, to be kind to myself and to finally work through all those stagnant pushed down feelings I was running away from for so long. I suppose I could say it's an enlightenment I have experienced. I still don't fit in but I'm at peace with that and realize that being unique is not a source of shame but a well of creativity and freedom.

*

DAWN WOINOVICK
Dawn was diagnosed with depression, posttraumatic stress disorder, degenerative disc disease at age 37, and a pituitary tumor at age 52

I believe the blessings I have received from my loss of health are to value myself and my health as a priority, to be able to better love and care for those around me. Also finding out where I fit into others' lives and who really values me as a person, as opposed to what people get from me or need me to do for them. Seeing the silver lining is really such a blessing because it helps you make the most of your time, which you come to understand is quite valuable.

CHAPTER EIGHTEEN

OUR HOPE

Be like the birds, sing after every storm.
-BETH MENDE CONNY

Hope is the fuel that propels us forward, urges us to get out of bed each morning. It is the promise that tomorrow will be better than today. Each breath we take and each footprint we leave is a measure of hope. So is hope possible in the face of lifelong health challenges?

*

CHRISTINE BASTONE
Christine became ill with chronic
fatigue syndrome at the age of 27

Hope is when you believe that somehow, someway, things will get better someday. Hope is also the knowledge that one day can change everything. It can be for the worse, or for the better. When I lost my health, of course it was for the worse. I have hope that one day things will change for the better.

I feel that hope is also wanting to see how everything turns out. It is living out the saying, "Where there is life, there is hope." And not wanting to exit, so to speak, right before things get better!

*

JERED DETWILER
Jered was diagnosed with a rare liver disorder,
Glycogen Storage Disease type 1a, as an infant
and hepatocellular cancer with liver tumors at age 31

Hope to me is knowing I can sit down with those I love for years to come and enjoy their company.

*

BONNIE FORSHEY
Bonnie was diagnosed with hepatitis C at age 41, rheumatoid and
osteoarthritis at age 48, diabetes and systemic lupus at age 50,
and Graves' disease and MAC disease at age 60

When I was diagnosed with chronic hepatitis C, there was no cure and it was pretty much a death sentence. I have lived with it for thirty-five years, and there is finally a treatment available with a high cure rate. I have hope for the future now. I will be free of this parasite that has been slowly killing me. I will have my energy back, be able to get out of bed, and also be able to return to work. I am looking forward to having quality time with my family and making good memories with my grandsons. I will not be remembered as the sick grandmother who was always in bed, and could not do anything. I have been given a second chance at life and will not waste another day of it.

*

VICKI HECKROTH
Vicki was diagnosed with rheumatoid
arthritis and fibromyalgia at age 45

Hope means to me that there will come a day when I will no longer feel not only the pain of being sick but that all of the tears and sadness will be wiped from this earth. Maybe even find a cure or better medication for my diseases. That I will once again be able to show affection and give hugs to my family that I love so dearly.

*

BRENDA L. KLEINSASSER
Brenda was diagnosed with rheumatoid arthritis at age 31
and a right frontal lobe meningioma brain tumor at age 48

Hope is one of my favorite words in the English language. It is something I cling to every day. Hope has gotten me through some very rough times. Hope allows me to continue to fight every day. If it were not for hope, I would have given up a long time ago. I strive to spread awareness and along with that I always include hope in the broad spectrum. Hope assures me that the sun will shine again during the dark days and storms of my life. Hope sustains me when the pain gets too much to bear at times. I always imagine what it will be like, once that attack on my body is over. That is hope personified. Writing about my challenges gives me hope. Finding those people who truly understand what it means to face challenges with such grace gives me hope. Hope is comfort when the tears are streaming down my face. Sometimes it hurts to feel so deeply, but hope reminds me that it will not always be this way. Hope allows me to move forward and make a difference every single day.

*

MARLISE MAGNA
Marlise was diagnosed with epilepsy in 1996, fibromyalgia and insulin resistance in 2009, and posttraumatic stress disorder in 2014

The bible states there is ALWAYS hope, faith and love. Hope to me means things can only get better and that this too shall pass.

*

LAYNE MARTIN
Layne was diagnosed with
psoriatic arthritis at age 47

Hope is being thankful and appreciating each day. I never know how I'm going to feel from day to day, so I'm just thankful when I have a good day and hope for more good days in the future.

I am also hopeful with modern medicine and science that someday soon a prevention and/or cure will be found for autoimmune diseases, cancer, heart disease and other health related diseases that now plague the world.

*

DENISE PURCELL
Denise was diagnosed with fibromyalgia
and degenerative disc disease at age 45

Hope is a possibility. That is a broad spectrum, I know. But if you don't at least have hope then there is nothing positive to focus on. And possibilities are endless like love. One hope at a time.

*

MARYELLEN ROACH
MaryEllen was diagnosed
with fibromyalgia at age 30

For me, hope is the same as faith. Hope is believing that God will make a way for things to be better. What causes fibromyalgia is currently unknown, and there is no cure at this time either. I truly and deeply hope answers will be found which will lead to a cure for not only fibromyalgia sufferers, but also for people who suffer from other related illnesses.

*

STACY ROORDA
Stacy was diagnosed with
metastatic breast cancer at age 37

"Now faith is the substance of things hoped for, the evidence of things not seen." Hebrews 11:1. The hope of the gospel is my hope, because without it we wouldn't have everlasting life. Just the fact that I know I'll be with my loved ones forever is what gets me out of bed in the morning and helps me enjoy each day. When I'm gone my family knows it's temporary until they join me, there's solace in that for all of us.

160

*

LAUREN VANDAL
Lauren suffered a traumatic
brain injury at age 35

Hope has been my savior throughout all of this. Even when I was at rock bottom there was something still inside me that wanted to keep going. Something that kept me waking up every morning and thinking THIS is the day it changes.

I can't really define hope. It was an invisible fire that burned inside me. I now realize just how strong I am, how my capacity to heal myself and others is huge. Hope has enabled me to take what happened and use it as a foundation for building something new. I still have days when hope is the only thing I have, days when the road of recovery takes a downturn. Hope is not something I acquired, it just "was." It was an in-built tool that rose to the challenge when I needed it the most.

*

DAWN WOINOVICK
Dawn was diagnosed with depression, posttraumatic stress disorder,
degenerative disc disease at age 37, and a pituitary tumor at age 52

Hope is believing in each moment and living each moment as if it is the only one that you have. Value it, putting quality into everything you do because each moment counts. This life is not just a cruise but a journey to be enjoyed. It is also a responsibility to give of yourself and receive what others have to share with you. That is what gives hope in the journey's final destination being a grand finale.

The wish for healing has always been half of health.
LUCIUS ANNAEUS SENECA

*

CHAPTER NINETEEN

OUR JOURNEY

Be soft. Do not let the world make you hard. Do not let
the pain make you hate. Do not let bitterness steal your
sweetness. -KURT VONNEGUT

Every journey is as unique as one's fingerprint, for we experience
different beliefs, different desires, different needs, different
tolerances, and often we walk different roads. Though we may not
see anyone else on the path, we are never truly alone for more walk
behind, beside, and in front of us. In this chapter lies the writers'
answers to the final question posed: What would you like the world
to know about your journey?

*

CHRISTINE BASTONE
Christine became ill with chronic
fatigue syndrome at the age of 27

What I would like the world to know is that just because I look
fine, doesn't necessarily mean I am fine. And that when you don't
believe me when I say I'm not fine, you invalidate me. Just because
you can't see something doesn't mean that it doesn't exist. Illness,
disease and chronic health problems are not always visible. You
have absolutely no idea how often I have come so close to envying
someone who has something like cancer. Simply because that is

something that people believe in. At least after the diagnosis, it is usually something you can see. If you see someone park in a disabled spot who looks fine, if they have the sticker, please give them the benefit of the doubt. Many people who legitimately have such stickers don't use them because of how they get treated when they do. That is very sad.

Rest is not a dirty word. Contrary to popular belief, things like rest, sleep, and taking care of yourself are important and smart, not selfish and lazy! Sometimes you can't "just do it." Oh, my how I hate that slogan! Trust me, if it was that easy, I would have figured it out by now. If I never pushed myself, I wouldn't get anything done. But I am very careful not to push too hard. Pushing harder is not the magical answer that society thinks it is. And I can't help but wonder how all the pushing of our kids in school is going to affect the health of those kids when they grow up.

Chronic fatigue is not all in my head. I'm not crazy, I'm not making it up, and I'm not faking being sick. Society's disbelief only makes things harder for me.

Oh, and I won't feel better if I exercise! No, not even going for a walk. Unfortunately exercise actually brings on my symptoms. I don't feel a rush of endorphins, it does not make me feel less depressed, and it won't help me get in shape if I can't get out of bed for the next three days!

I also do not just need to get out of the house! I have to be out of the house too much as it is. When I can stay home, I take advantage of it. I am a homebody, I actually like to be home most of the time. I guess I'm kind of funny that way. And on the odd occasion when these four walls start closing in on me...I have a car, and a driver's license, and so I am perfectly capable of going somewhere if I need to do so.

In January 2002, I came across this wonderful chronic fatigue glossary. I found it online, and I printed it. The only reason that I can tell you when I printed it, is that the date I printed it is on it! I wish I could tell you who wrote it. But all I have is the website that I got it from. I would put that here, but of course it doesn't exist anymore. Anyway, there are a few definitions that I really agreed with and liked. I'll give you the best two:

- Honorary Degree in Logistics And Planning: Should be awarded to every person with chronic fatigue syndrome who achieves anything at all in three years of illness.

- Superheroes: Well people who jump tall buildings. CFS sufferers who get out of bed in the morning (by the way, CFS stands for chronic fatigue syndrome).

I'm going to end this with a few definitions of my own:

- 2000: About how old I feel.
- Getting out of bed: Major accomplishment.
- Staying out of bed: Even bigger accomplishment.
- Exhausted: Not a strong enough word for how I feel.
- Tired: What I wish I felt.
- Piece of cake: What nothing is anymore.
- Exercise: Something I can't do very often anymore.
- Out of shape: Something I am mostly because I so rarely exercise.
- Okay: Answer to the question, "How are you?" which is usually much closer to the truth than "fine" or "good."
- Hit by a truck: How I feel most of the time, but still better than the stretched out rubber band feeling that I try very hard to avoid.
- I'm not feeling very well: Phrase that even I'm very tired of hearing.
- Purple Heart: Medal that should be awarded to anyone with CFS.

*

JERED DETWILER
Jered was diagnosed with a rare liver disorder,
Glycogen Storage Disease type 1a, as an infant
and hepatocellular cancer with liver tumors at age 31

Living with a disease all your life can be rough. Some dreams you may have had can be crushed. Those around you may not understand or want to understand the disease and problems you live with. Other unexpected benefits such as traveling around and having a wish granted through the Make-A-Wish organization can definitely be counted as a highlight more so than what other people get to do.

*

BONNIE FORSHEY
Bonnie was diagnosed with hepatitis C at age 41, rheumatoid and
osteoarthritis at age 48, diabetes and systemic lupus at age 50,
and Graves' disease and MAC disease at age 60

I was always a very strong, independent woman. I worked full-time, raised two children, and put myself through nursing school. I contracted chronic hepatitis C when I was a student nurse via a blood splash from a sick patient thirty-five years ago. I continued to work until ten years ago, and had to go on disability because I could not function any longer. I became so weak and so tired that I could actually go to sleep standing up. I could no longer even drive a car. I became bedbound and felt like a geriatric patient. It is very difficult to give up your independence, your financial stability and your dignity. The HCV really wreaked havoc with my immune system, and opened the door for more diseases. Eventually, I had problems breathing, due to asthma and MAC disease. I have severe joint pain, due to rheumatoid arthritis and lupus, and debilitating fatigue. I was diagnosed with hypothyroidism, osteoporosis, diabetes, congestive heart failure, hypertension, GERD and gastroparesis. I lost my appetite and was unable to keep anything down. Every system in my body was affected, and I felt so close to death. It has been a terrible journey, but it is almost over. I have a second chance at life, and I will not take anything for granted.

*

VICKI HECKROTH
Vicki was diagnosed with rheumatoid
arthritis and fibromyalgia at age 45

I want people to know that the pain is real. That none of us just decided to one day wake up and say, "From now on I am going to pretend to be sick with an autoimmune disease so that I can get some powerful meds." That we are not addicts. We do not take the medication to get high or even to change our thinking. We take them because without them we would most likely not be able to get through the day. I also want others to know that we don't pretend to not feel well just to avoid you. We would give anything to be able to hang out and have fun. That just isn't the cards for us much any longer.

*

BRENDA L. KLEINSASSER
Brenda was diagnosed with rheumatoid arthritis at age 31
and a right frontal lobe meningioma brain tumor at age 48

Being a brain tumor survivor is a complex sort of life. You will not truly understand it unless you have actually been through it. There are emotions so deep and strong that at times they are scary to deal with. I also count these as blessings, as they have caused me to possess much more empathy. I would like to be able to express what I am feeling without that fear of judgment. What I mean by that is, allow me to be exactly who I am at any given moment. I need to be able to work through all types of emotions. I really want to be a part of this whole thing called life.

I know my personality has changed, but that is not my fault. I cannot control what has happened deep inside my brain. I can only try to control how I deal with it. It would be much easier if I were given the freedom to just be ME. I have a lot to offer. Give me a chance to show you what I can do. I have ideas and feelings too. I have a lot to bring to the table. Please give me the courtesy to do so.

With my rheumatoid arthritis, there will be days when it is too difficult to perform some tasks. On those days, I would just ask that you possess a little understanding. My pain is with me pretty much twenty-four hours a day, but I have to continue to fight. My pain or my disease is unique and not like anyone else's. Please stop comparing it to your friend or relative. You have no idea what I go through on a daily basis to survive. I want to continue to inspire others. With both of these challenges, I have a lot to offer as I know firsthand what it is like to live with a chronic illness and also the challenges of being a brain tumor survivor. I want to be allowed to be involved in sharing that with others. As I said before, I have a lot to bring to the table. I am very experienced when it comes to medical challenges. I have had almost twenty procedures myself, so I am very familiar with hospitals. I want to continue to be able to speak out for those who feel they have no voice. Consider me someone who has your back.

The one thing I really want to bring home is to be patient with me. I am trying the best I can every day. Some days are truly difficult to even think clearly, as pain can cause brain fog. I also have that extra challenge now with being a brain tumor survivor. I sometimes mix details up, so I really have to evaluate something real carefully before I continue with the next step. Both of these challenges are real tough at times to deal with, but I know that I possess the strength and fortitude to do so. When I was diagnosed with rheumatoid arthritis in 1991, I thought my life was over. It is clearly not so. When I was diagnosed with my brain tumor and had my craniotomy in 2008, I had no idea that my life would change forever. My battles and blessings continue to intersect and bring hope to me personally every day of my life.

*

*

MARLISE MAGNA
Marlise was diagnosed with epilepsy in 1996, fibromyalgia and
insulin resistance in 2009, and posttraumatic stress disorder in 2014

I've learnt to take things slowly - ten minutes at a time if I must. Even though at times it feels like there is no hope and your life is over, time does heal. Also - love is everything and a small smile or act of kindness helps you feel better. Most of all, have no expectations. Hope for the best, expect the worst, and you will end up somewhere in between. Also - rest as much as you need to. Be kind to yourself, spoil yourself. And if you need to do what you need to do regarding taking medication, do it. Most importantly, do your research on what treatments help.

*

LAYNE MARTIN
Layne was diagnosed with
psoriatic arthritis at age 47

Loss of health is a constant worry and sometimes it consumes your every thought. You tend to get tunnel vision as you're so focused on yourself that you forget to include others in your life. It's very self-absorbing as you either start to exclude those around you that love you, or you overcompensate and expect them to do everything for you. It's a hard road to walk as you try to find balance so you can maintain healthy relationships as you struggle to stay afloat. I continue to volunteer and use my knowledge as a patient advocate. Some days it's from my recliner in my living room with my laptop but I hope that I can continue to help others by sharing what resources I know and advocating for better health care.

*

DENISE PURCELL
Denise was diagnosed with fibromyalgia
and degenerative disc disease at age 45

I would like the world to know that I am disabled. That doesn't mean I'm a lower status of a person. I don't get everything free. And although I do get some medical help, most times it is embarrassing for me because help means to a lot of people lazy or lying. Most people who need care don't get it because the medical doctors only take certain insurances. I worked for a good many years and then chose to become a stay-at-home mom. But there are no benefits for that except from your children's heart.

*

MARYELLEN ROACH
MaryEllen was diagnosed
with fibromyalgia at age 30

When I was first diagnosed with fibromyalgia, I didn't realize it could and would get worse. I didn't realize what an enormous impact it could and would have on my life. I didn't realize how depressing and limiting this disease would be. I didn't realize how misunderstood fibromyalgia truly is and I also didn't realize how many symptoms I've had that initially weren't listed as fibro symptoms. I frequently learn how one of my "quirks" actually stem from a fibro symptom.

Lastly, I didn't realize how cruel people could be about an illness that isn't visible on the outside. I would like everyone to know that fibromyalgia is very real. Even if fibromyalgia and other invisible disease sufferers don't look sick, it is not a made-up condition or an excuse used to get out of doing anything, the illness is just on the inside. Most people with a disease like this would absolutely love to have even one symptom-free day to do the things they need and want to do, feel accomplished, feel comfort and actually be able to obtain rest.

I've seen pictures that try to show what fibromyalgia would look like if it was visible on the outside. The particular picture I'm thinking of shows a person's back covered in horrible looking bruises with veins and pressure points colored purple and bruised as well. That picture is pretty accurate, although I would add flames to the muscles. I think most people would be horrified if they could truly see how it feels.

Mostly, I want other fibromyalgia and invisible disease sufferers to know they are not alone. There are other people in this world who relate and fully believe your never-ending struggles. I want the people who can wake up without excruciating pain, who can sit comfortably, who can do whatever they want without worrying about the pain value, extreme fatigue or other symptoms, to recognize and appreciate what they have.

I want the world to be kinder and more understanding toward others. I love the saying, "Be kind, for everyone is fighting a hard battle." That saying is just so accurate and something all of us need to keep in mind. The Bible also tells us to treat others the same way we want to be treated. I don't think that could be put any simpler.

*

STACY ROORDA
Stacy was diagnosed with
metastatic breast cancer at age 37

It really did show me what I'm made of and how strong I really am. Also, I want others to know that my story is a part of me but doesn't define who I am. I've been asked to help out with cancer walks, pro-life issues and a handful of other causes but I really don't have the desire to do so. By saying I chose not to terminate my pregnancy and using that as a platform to voice my opinions, or helping others voice theirs, just feels wrong to me. It was just such a personal and emotionally devastating time that to try to piece it apart isn't possible. There was nothing heroic about the decision to stay pregnant because to Matt and I, it wasn't a decision at all. In fact we never even discussed the idea. I know he would have been fine with whatever I decided but I just never even felt the need to bring it up. One day I was diagnosed with the cancer and the next day I was told I was pregnant. To me being pregnant meant that I had another child to protect, protect with my life if necessary, just like I would protect my other kids.

The next month after my diagnosis at Christmas, Matt bought me a beautiful diamond necklace and pearl bracelet with the signature pink ribbon on them. I knew it meant so much for Matt, it was a way he felt like he could help because he felt so helpless. I've never ever worn them and don't think I ever can. It's just such a small part of who I am and quite honestly I don't want to spend my day talking about cancer, it's depressing! There are plenty of people who do wear those things and that's okay too. Whatever brings someone comfort is so important and so necessary in times of trauma and sadness.

*

LAUREN VANDAL
Lauren suffered a traumatic
brain injury at age 35

Loss of any kind is devastating. It cuts a furrow through the middle of your life and casts aside joy, love, safety and permanence. It is something ANYONE can experience at any time. BUT, little by little, piece by piece we get through it. It makes us cry, it makes us feel weak, it sometimes even makes us laugh. We take the scattered bits of our souls and glue them back together and where the scar appears we are stronger. The vulnerability and pain we experience with loss are our greatest allies. We don't realize it at the time but they are there to guide us through the dark and show us the way back to ourselves. Listen to them, they are wise. Embrace the dark as well as the light, there are lessons in both. Don't run away from the night because without it there is no sunrise.

You WILL get through this. You WILL discover parts of yourself you never knew were there and as my friend always tells me, "You don't need fixing, you are not broken."

*

DAWN WOINOVICK
Dawn was diagnosed with depression, posttraumatic stress disorder, degenerative disc disease at age 37, and a pituitary tumor at age 52

I have experienced a great deal of loss on my journey thus far, but my health issues has been by far the most challenging. To lose your ability to do certain things or getting confused very easily, having your mind know what to say and the words not come out. Being an intelligent woman and having others look or talk behind your back as if you're not all there, and there is nothing you can do to get yourself better. That can get you very depressed on occasion, if you let it. But you must ALWAYS remember you are a vessel with a heart, soul and spirit and you have a God who made you just the way you are.

You are not your sickness or your health problems. They don't make you. YOU are fearfully and wonderfully made, and one day we will all be whole again, so hang in there with me my friend. We can get through this together.

*Hope is being able to see that there is light
despite all of the darkness.*
DESMOND TUTU

*

CHAPTER TWENTY

FINDING THE SUNRISE

One night in my own journey through loss, I had one of *those* dreams: a vivid nightmare that stays with you. I was running westward in a frantic attempt to catch the setting sun as it descended below the horizon. Rapidly advancing from behind was nightfall; foreboding and frightening, it was a pitch black abyss. And it was coming directly for me. I ran desperately, as fast as my legs could go, toward the sunset, but my attempt was futile; it descended below the horizon, out of my reach. Oh, the looming nightfall was terrifying! But it was clear that if I wanted to ever see the sun again, I had to stop running west and, instead, turn around and walk east to begin my journey through the great murky abyss, the nightfall of grief. For just as there would be no rainbow without the rain, the sun only rises on the other side of night. The message was clear: it was futile to avoid my grief; I had to allow it to swallow me whole. Then, and only then, would I find my way through it and out the other side.

Our journeys might be different, but grief comes in many forms. When we lose our health or receive a devastating diagnosis, it can take our breath away. And it's only natural to grieve what shall be no more. And so I share this chapter in all Grief Diaries titles, because it can be helpful regardless of one's loss.

I once read in a bereavement book that if we don't allow ourselves to experience the full scope of our loss, it will come back to bite us. After losing our teenage daughter in a car accident, I couldn't fathom how it could possibly get any worse. But I didn't want to test that theory, and so I gave in and allowed my grief to swallow me whole. I allowed myself to wail on my daughter's bedroom floor. I penned my deep emotions, regardless of who might read it. I created a national radio show to openly and candidly discuss our journeys with anyone who wanted to call in. And I allowed myself to sink to the bottom of the fiery pits of hell. This, in turn, lit a fire under me, so to speak, to find a way out.

Today, I'm often asked how I manage my grief so well. Some assume that because I have found peace and joy, I'm simply avoiding my grief. Others believe that because I work in the bereavement field, I'm wallowing in self-pity. Well, which is it?

Neither. I will miss my child with every breath I take. Just like you, I will always have my moments. But I have also found purpose, beauty and joy again. It takes hard work and determination to overcome any kind of loss, and it also takes the ability to let go and succumb to the journey. Do not be afraid of the tears, sorrow, and heartbreak; they are a natural reaction, and are imperative to your healing.

As you walk your own path, avail yourself to whatever tools that might ease your discomfort, for each one was created by someone who walked in your shoes and understands the heartache. While there are many wonderful bereavement resources available, what brings comfort to one person might irritate the next. Bereavement tools are not one-size-fits-all, so if one tool doesn't work, find another.

Lastly, grief is not something we get "over," like a mountain. Rather, it is something we get "through," like the rapids of Niagara Falls. Without the kayak and paddle. And plenty of falls. But it's also survivable. And if others have survived this journey, why not me? And why not you?

On the following pages are the baby steps I took to find balance again in life. They took great effort at first, lots of patience with myself, and the gentle understanding that life will never be what it once was. But like any dedicated routine, these baby steps got easier over time, and the reward of finding balance in my life worth it.

1. VALIDATING OUR EMOTIONS

The first step is to validate your emotions. When we talk about our grief, we aren't ruminating in our sorrow or feeling sorry for ourselves. By discussing it, we are actually processing it. If we aren't allowed to process it, then it becomes silent grief. Silent grief is deadly grief.

Find a friend who will patiently listen while you discuss your loss for fifteen minutes every day. Set the timer, and ask them not to say anything during those fifteen minutes. Explain that it is important for you to just ramble without interruption, guidance, or judgment. You need not have the same listener each time, but practice this step <u>every</u> day.

2. COMPASSIONATE THOUGHTS

Find yourself a quiet spot. It can be your favorite chair, in your car, in your office, or even in your garden. Then clear your head and for five minutes think nothing but compassionate thoughts about yourself. Not your spouse, not your children, not your coworkers, but yourself.

Having trouble? Fill in the blanks below, and then give yourself permission to really validate those positive qualities. Do this every day.

I have a _____

Example: good heart, gentle soul, witty personality

I make a _____

Example: good lasagna, potato salad, scrapbook, quilt

I'm a good_____

Example: friend, gardener, knitter, painter, poem writer

People would say I'm _____

Example: funny, kind, smart, gentle, generous, humble, creative

3. TENDER LOVING CARE

While grieving, it is important to consider yourself in the intensive care unit of Grief United Hospital, and treat accordingly. How would nurses treat you if you were their patient in the ICU? They would be compassionate, gentle, and allow for plenty of rest. That is exactly how you should treat yourself. Also, consider soothing your physical self with TLC as an attentive way to honor your emotional pain. This doesn't mean you have to book an expensive massage. If wearing fuzzy blue socks offers a smidgen of comfort, then wear them unabashedly. If whipped cream on your cocoa offers a morsel of pleasure, then indulge unapologetically.

Treating our five senses to anything that offers a perception of delight might not erase the emotional heartache, but it will offer a reminder that not all pleasure is lost. List five ways you can offer yourself tender loving care, and then incorporate at least three into your day, every day. With practice, the awareness of delight eventually becomes effortless, and is an important step toward regaining joy.

TLC suggestions:

- Shower or bathe with a lovely scented soap
- Soak in a warm tub with Epsom salts or a splash of bath oil
- Wear a pair of extra soft socks
- Light a fragrant candle
- Listen to relaxing music
- Apply a rich lotion to your skin before bed
- Indulge in a few bites of your favorite treat
- Enjoy a mug of your favorite soothing herbal tea
- Add whipped cream to a steaming mug of cocoa
- _____
- _____
- _____
- _____

4. SEE THE BEAUTY

Listening to the birds outside my bedroom window every morning was something I had loved since childhood. But when Aly died, I found myself deaf and blind to the beauty around me. My world had become colorless and silent. On one particular morning as I struggled to get out of bed, I halfheartedly noticed the birds chirping outside my bedroom window. My heart sank as I realized that they had been chirping all along, but I was now deaf to their morning melody. Panic set in as I concluded that I would never enjoy life's beauty ever again. Briefly entertaining suicide to escape the profound pain, I quickly ruled it out. My family had been through so much already, I couldn't dump further pain on them. But in order to survive the heartbreak, I had to find a way to allow beauty back into my life.

So on that particular morning as I lay in bed, I forced myself to listen and really *hear* the birds. Every morning from that point forward, I repeated that same exercise. With persistent practice, it became easier and then eventually effortless to appreciate the birds' chirping and singsongs. Glorious beauty and sounds have once again returned to my world.

Profound grief can appear to rob our world of all beauty. Yet the truth is, and despite our suffering, beauty continues to surround us. The birds continue to sing, flowers continue to bloom, the surf continues to ebb and flow. Reconnecting to our surroundings helps us to reintegrate back into our environment.

Begin by acknowledging one small pleasantry each day. Perhaps your ears register the sound of singing birds. Or you catch the faint scent of warm cookies as you walk past a bakery. Or notice the sun's illumination of a nearby red rosebush. Give yourself permission to notice one pleasantry, and allow it to *really* register.

Here are some suggestions:

- Listen to the birds sing (hearing)
- Observe pretty cloud formations (sight)
- Visit a nearby park and listen to the children (hearing)
- Notice the pretty colors of blooming flowers (sight)
- Light a fragrant candle (scent)
- See the beauty in the sunset (sight)
- Attend a local recital, concert, play, or comedy act (hearing)
- Wear luxury socks (touch)
- Wrap yourself in a soft scarf or sweater (touch)
- Indulge in whipped cream on your cocoa (taste)
- Enjoy a Hershey's chocolate kiss (taste)

5. PROTECT YOUR HEALTH

After our daughter's accident I soon found myself fighting an assortment of viruses including head colds, stomach flus, sore throats and more, compounding my already frazzled emotions. Studies show that profound grief throws our body into "flight or fight" syndrome for months and months, which is very hard on our physical body. Thus, it becomes critical to guard our physical health. Incorporating a few changes into our daily routine feels hard at first, but soon gets easy. Plus, a stronger physical health helps to strengthen our coping skills.

Below are a few suggestions to consider adding to your daily routine to help your physical self withstand the emotional upheaval.

- Practice good sleep hygiene
- Drink plenty of water
- Take a short walk outside every day
- Resist simple carbohydrates (I'm a food addict, so I know that avoiding simple carbs is worth its weight in gold)
- Keep a light calendar and guard your time carefully, don't allow others to dictate and overflow your schedule

6. FIND AN OUTLET

For a long time in the grief journey, everything is painful. In the early days, just getting out of bed and taking a shower can be exhausting. Housecleaning, grocery shopping, and routine errands often take a backseat or disappear altogether. As painful as it is, it's very important to find an outlet that gets you out of bed each day. Finding something to distract you from the pain, occupy your mind, and soothe your senses can be tricky, but possible. Performing a repetitive action can calm your mood, and even result in a new craft or gifts to give.

Beginning a new outlet may feel exhausting at first, just remember that the first step is always the hardest. And you don't have to do it forever, just focus on it for the time being.

Possible activities include:

- Learn to mold chocolate or make soap
- Learn how to bead, knit, crochet, or quilt
- Volunteer at a local shelter
- Learn a new sport such as golf or kayaking
- Create a memorial garden in a forgotten part of the yard
- Join Pinterest
- Doodle or draw
- Mold clay
- Learn to scrapbook
- Join a book club

Loss of health can be hell. But when walking through hell, your only option is to keep going. Eventually the dark night fades to dawn, and the sun begins its ascent once again. Just keep going and you, too, will find the sunrise.

Lynda Cheldelin Fell

One smile can change a day.
One hug can change a life
One hope can change a destiny.
LYNDA CHELDELIN FELL

*

SURVIVING LOSS OF HEALTH

MEET THE WRITERS

There's a bright future for you at every turn,
even if you miss one.

*

*

CHRISTINE BASTONE
Christine became ill with chronic fatigue syndrome at the age of 27
C.Bastone@mail.com   *   www.facebook.com/CricketsPlace1

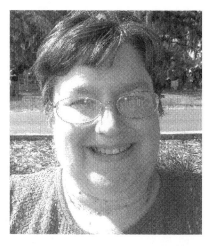

Christine Bastone is a stay-at-home mom in her forties who has only recently figured out that she wants to be a writer when she grows up! She was born in northeast Ohio and moved to Florida in May 1995. She married Angelo Bastone in July 1997. They have a son, Joshua, born in 2001 and a daughter, Katelyn, born in 2004. The four of them live together in their house at the end of a quiet street in central Florida.

Christine has always loved to read, and was thrilled when her husband gave her a Kindle for Christmas in 2011. She has since read hundreds of Kindle books. Christine is co-author of *Grief Diaries: Loss of a Sibling*, and contributed to the book, *Faces of Suicide, Volume 1*, available on Amazon as a Kindle book. She has also been a guest on Grief Diaries Radio twice in 2014, both episodes are available on iTunes. At the time of this publication she is working on a new book called, *Advice from Tomorrow*.

*

JERED DETWILER
Jered was diagnosed with a rare liver disorder,
Glycogen Storage Disease type 1a, as an infant
and hepatocellular cancer with liver tumors at age 31

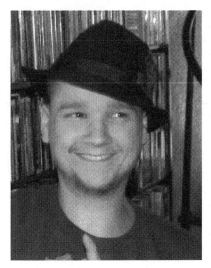

Jered Detwiler was born and raised in the Seattle area. He has an older brother who he enjoys spending time with. Jered lives with his parents, a sister and his cat Smokey.

His dream was to go into the military following high school but having Glycogen Storage Disease prevented him from doing so. Jered currently works for a local screen printing company.

*

BONNIE FORSHEY
Bonnie was diagnosed with hepatitis C at age 41
rheumatoid and osteoarthritis at age 48
diabetes and systemic lupus at age 50
Graves' disease and MAC disease at age 60
bonnieforshey@msn.com

Bonnie Forshey was born in Lewistown, Pennsylvania, and raised in New Castle, Delaware. She later moved to Swainsboro, Georgia, where she attended Emanuel County Junior College. She earned the Science Merit Award and graduated with her A.S. degree. Later she attended Gordon State College in Barnesville, Georgia, earning a B.S. in Nursing.

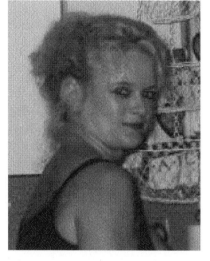

Bonnie spent most of her life working in medical-surgical, geriatrics, rehabilitation and long-term care facilities. Bonnie also raised two children, and worked as a nursing assistant, unit secretary, and in Medical Records while putting herself through school. Bonnie has two grandsons and currently resides in both Port Royal, Pennsylvania, and Brandon, Florida.

*

VICKI HECKROTH
Vicki was diagnosed with
rheumatoid arthritis and fibromyalgia at age 45

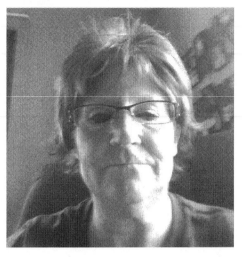

Vicki was born in Spencer, Iowa. She received her early education in Worthington, Minnesota. In fifth grade she moved to Greenville, Iowa and attended school at Clay Central until she graduated in 1979.

Upon graduation Vicki married her high school sweetheart to which three children were born. They divorced eight years later due to domestic abuse. She then dated a man for two years who also abused her.

Vicki has been married to her husband Tim for over twenty-five years. He is a good husband and treats her children as if they are his own. Vicki worked for several years as head waitress for Family Table in Spencer, Iowa, and then as general manager for Burger King in Storm Lake, Iowa, until becoming disabled in 2011.

*

BRENDA L. KLEINSASSER
Brenda was diagnosed with rheumatoid arthritis at age 31
and a right frontal lobe meningioma brain tumor at age 48
http://brendasbrainstorm.blogspot.com

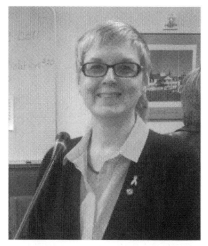

Brenda Kleinsasser resides in Bismarck, North Dakota, the capital city. She has worked in various avenues of the medical field for over thirty years. She was editor of the CreakyJoints Poet's Corner (& Artists too) for three years, a unique online publication where the emphasis is on encouraging those who live with a chronic illness to allow their creativity to shine.

She is also a fierce patient advocate for both brain tumors and rheumatoid arthritis, as she has also lived with RA for over twenty-four years. Her stance on advocacy is speaking up for those who cannot, or feel they have no voice. She has testified to that end in her own state of North Dakota, representing the patient's voice. In her spare time, she enjoys writing her blog, Brenda's Brainstorm and Trevor, a golden retriever who is her storyteller and helper with spreading awareness and hope. She also enjoys journaling and singing.

*

MARLISE MAGNA
Marlise was diagnosed with epilepsy in 1996
fibromyalgia and insulin resistance in 2009
and posttraumatic stress disorder in 2014

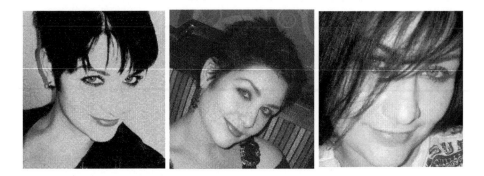

Marlise was born December 2, 1978, in Johannesburg, South Africa and is the first of two children. Her life has been nothing but out of the ordinary as most people would describe it. She studied drama at South Africa's National School of the Arts before becoming a Jill of all trades. She's worked as a canine behaviorist, wedding planner, TV presenter, matchmaker and dance instructor, to name a few. At age thirty-five, after two divorces and many suicide attempts, she finally found what she wanted to do and is currently studying to become a pastor. She has been instrumental in planting two churches involved in relationship counseling, praise and worship singing. She is also lead singer in her own Christian band.

Marlise is also director of an alternative clothing and interior design company, magazine editor, and proofreader. Marlise is an avid reader and loves nothing better than doing research and trivia games. Standup comedy and watching reality TV series is another favorite pastime. She lives with her mom and her beloved dog, Juke.

*

DEANA MARTIN

Deana was diagnosed with chronic depression and anxiety disorder at
age 26, breast cancer at age 33, and posttraumatic stress disorder at
age 45 after losing both children in a car accident
deana@cryformenomore.com * www.cryformenomore.com

Deana Martin is a childless
parent who lost her only two
children in a tragic auto accident
in 2011. Miraculously Deana
was spared her only granddaughter who was in the car
behind them. Since the death of
her children Deana has become
a certified grief specialist and
has channeled the love for her
children to other families facing
loss.

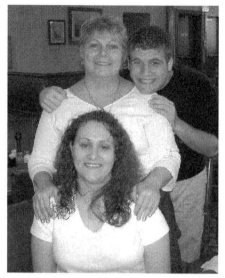

Before this tragedy, Deana was
a project manager in the
pharmaceutical industry and had enjoyed a twenty-five-year career
with several fortune 500 pharmaceutical companies starting with
Eli Lilly in 1988, the year her son was born. Deana has faced many
adversities in life and feels each one makes her stronger. Deana is a
breast cancer survivor, and is no stranger to trauma. She hopes to
help people heal by showing them how to find the strength and
courage needed along the journey.

Deana is co-founder and vice president of Cry For Me, No More, a
national nonprofit serving the bereaved, a founding board member
of National Grief & Hope Coalition, and co-author of *Grief Diaries:
Loss of a Child*.

*

LAYNE MARTIN
Layne was diagnosed with psoriatic arthritis at age 47

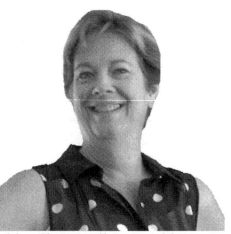

Layne Martin was born and raised in the beautiful Pacific Northwest. At a young age she was captivated by nurses. She loved everything about them, their crisp white dress uniforms, the white shoes and nylons, even the large white hats that they wore on their heads. Layne pursued a degree as a registered nurse and quickly gained the respect of fellow peers and physicians alike. She rapidly moved her way up the ranks and eventually she found her true passion working in emergency medicine.

As Layne continued to excel in her profession, she enjoyed mentoring those new to the emergency department. But at the age of 47, right in the peak of Layne's career, her world came crashing down when she was diagnosed with psoriatic arthritis, a destructive autoimmune disease. Soon she was plagued with the debilitating effects of the arthritis and was forced into early retirement, leaving a profession that she dearly loved and was destined to do.

Today, Layne volunteers her time writing blogs as a regional outreach manager and patient advocate for CreakyJoints. She also participates in the National Arthritis Database and recently was featured in an article in Everyday Health titled, "Managing Bad Days with Psoriatic Arthritis."

*

DENISE PURCELL
Denise was diagnosed with fibromyalgia
and degenerative disc disease at age 45
psunshine07@hotmail.com

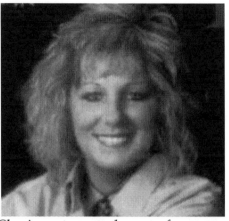

Denise Purcell was born in Syracuse, New York. The oldest of seven children, Denise became a mother at the early age of sixteen, and had five daughters by the time she was thirty-one.

Denise is an artist who has had artwork displayed in a few shows. She has also had some of her poems published. She is a strong advocate for many injustices that she herself has overcome and continues to do so. She is caring and trying to live her life according to her own truth. Her children have always been her world. She is proudly dealing with empty nest syndrome, with the last of her children now in college. Denise views life as a chance to see the beauty in adversity, and is trying to heal her broken heart since her daughter died in 2011.

*

MARYELLEN ROACH
MaryEllen was diagnosed with fibromyalgia at age 30

MaryEllen Roach was raised on a forty-acre farm in southern Illinois where her family raised sheep and other animals. MaryEllen graduated high school in 1996 with honors. She moved to St. Louis, Missouri, at the age of nineteen where she modeled and also worked for large companies based in St. Louis.

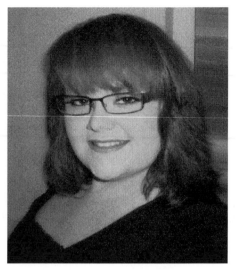

After the loss of her older sister and two young nieces, MaryEllen, her parents Marvin and Yvonna, her younger sister Ashley and Ashley's husband Moi all moved to northern California where they currently reside.

*

STACY ROORDA
Stacy was diagnosed with metastatic breast cancer at age 37

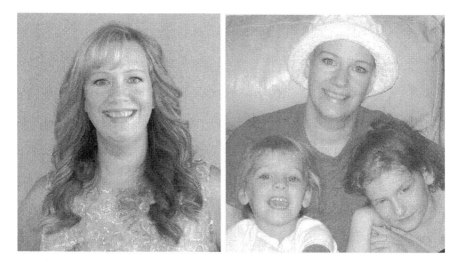

Stacy Roorda is the youngest of five children. After graduating from high school she briefly attended college but wanderlust soon took her on an eight-year adventure around the world. After settling back in her hometown, she met her future husband and they now live in Lynden, Washington, along with their three lively daughters.

Stacy is an international bestselling author, originally sharing her story, "Pregnant with Cancer," in *The Missing Piece: A Transformational Loss*. Her story has also been featured in TheBlaze as well as on Vimeo.

TheBlaze: http://www.theblaze.com/contributions/pregnant-with-stage-four-breast-cancer-she-believes-the-prayers-of-thousands-saved-her-and-her-child/

Vimeo: https://vimeo.com/82251139

*

LAUREN VANDAL
Lauren suffered a traumatic brain injury at age 35
braingirlandcat.wordpress.com

Lauren Vandal was born in Manchester, England but moved to Northern Ireland to start a new life in 2012. She particularly enjoys nature, animals, reading, meditating, walking and gardening.

Lauren lives with her partner and a fluffy bundle of a bunny named Groovy Bruce. They share a cottage in the beautiful countryside of County Down surrounded by sheep, cows and birds.

Lauren often dreams of being able to run up hills again and go for gorgeous meals.

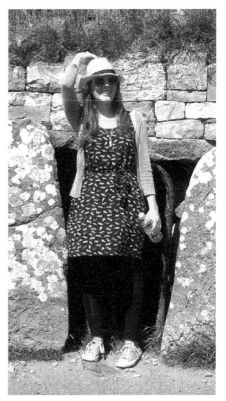

*

DAWN WOINOVICK
Dawn was diagnosed with depression, posttraumatic stress disorder, degenerative disc disease at age 37, and a pituitary tumor at age 52

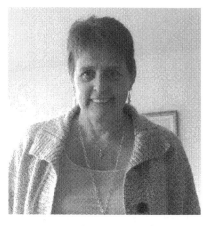

Dawn Woinovick is a mother of three grown children. She loves people and helping others any way she can, though she says that sometimes that's a problem because she trusts everyone and in today's world you need to have good discernment. She is a book reviewer for Amazon, CBD, GoodReads, and others and enjoys reading.

She considers herself a very spiritual person and believes in God, Jesus and the Holy Spirit. She believes that one only stops growing when they die. Dawn just became an ordained minister not affiliated with any one church, she goes where God calls. He often sends people to her. Dawn has helped in doing small groups on incest, sexual assault, domestic violence, and believes there is no true healing without God though Dawn is everyone's friend.

One laugh can scatter a hundred griefs.
LYNDA CHELDELIN FELL

*

THANK YOU

I am deeply indebted to the writers who contributed to *Grief Diaries: Surviving Loss of Health.* Such a collaboration sheds crucial insight into the daily challenges all of us face when diagnosed with lifelong health conditions. In doing so, we hope to offer comfort to those who find themselves on the same path.

I'm humbled to partner with my two sisters, Layne Martin, R.N. and Stacy Roorda, to bring this book project to fruition. I'm also grateful to author Annah Elizabeth for helping to draft paragraph introductions.

There simply are no words to express how much I love my husband Jamie, our children, and our wonderfully supportive family and friends for being there through laughter and tears, and encouraging me at every turn. None of this would have been possible without their unquestioning love that continues to surround me every moment.

Lynda Cheldelin Fell

Shared joy is doubled joy;
shared sorrow is half a sorrow.
SWEDISH PROVERB

*

ABOUT

LYNDA CHELDELIN FELL

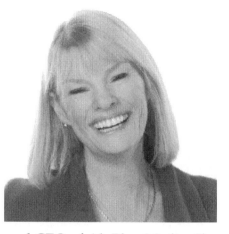

Considered a pioneer in the field of inspirational hope in the aftermath of loss, Lynda Cheldelin Fell has a passion for producing ground-breaking projects that create a legacy of help, healing, and hope. She is the creator of the 5-star anthology book series Grief Diaries, board president of the National Grief & Hope Coalition, and CEO of AlyBlue Media. She has interviewed Dr. Martin Luther King's daughter, Trayvon Martin's mother, sisters of the late Nicole Brown Simpson; Pastor Todd Burpo of Heaven is For Real, CNN commentator Dr. Ken Druck, and other societal newsmakers on finding healing and hope in the aftermath of life's harshest challenges.

Lynda's own story began in 2007, when she had an alarming dream about her young teenage daughter, Aly. In the dream, Aly was a backseat passenger in a car that veered off the road and sailed into a lake. Aly sank with the car, leaving behind an open book floating face down on the water. Two years later, Lynda's dream became reality when Aly was tragically killed as a backseat passenger in a car accident while coming home from a swim meet. Overcome with grief, Lynda's 46-year-old husband suffered a major stroke that left him with severe disabilities, traumatically changing the family dynamics yet again.

The following year, Lynda was invited to share her remarkable story about finding hope after loss, and she accepted. That cathartic experience inspired her to create ground-breaking projects spanning national events, radio, film and books to help others who share the same journey feel less alone.

In the aftermath of losing her daughter, Lynda discovered that helping others was a powerful way to heal her own heart. To her mind, one wounded soul extending compassion to another is the ultimate act of kindness. The Grief Diaries series was born and built on this belief.

Now one of the foremost grief experts in the United States, Lynda is dedicated to helping ordinary people share their own extraordinary stories of survival and hope in the aftermath of loss.

Because of that floating book her daughter left behind, Lynda now understands that the dream in 2007 was actually a glimpse into a divine plan destined to bring comfort, healing and hope to people around the world.

lynda@lyndafell.com | www.lyndafell.com | www.griefdiaries.com

ABOUT THE SERIES

It's important that we share our experiences with other people. Your story will heal you, and your story will heal somebody else. -IYANLA VANZANT

Grief Diaries is a series of anthology books exploring true stories about the life's challenges and losses. Created by international bestselling author and bereaved mother Lynda Cheldelin Fell, the series began with eight titles exploring unique losses shared by people around the world. Over a hundred people in six countries registered for those first eight titles, and the books were launched in December 2015. Following their release, organizations and individuals began asking Lynda to create additional titles to help raise awareness about their plights. To date, more than 300 writers are sharing their courageous stories in more than thirty anthology titles now in the works.

Now a 5-star series, a portion of profits from every book in the series goes to national organizations serving those in need.

Humanity's legacy of stories and storytelling is the most precious we have.
All wisdom is in our stories and songs.
DORIS LESSING

*

ALYBLUE MEDIA TITLES

PUBLISHED
Grief Diaries: Surviving Loss of a Spouse
Grief Diaries: Surviving Loss of a Child
Grief Diaries: Surviving Loss of a Sibling
Grief Diaries: Surviving Loss of a Parent
Grief Diaries: Surviving Loss of an Infant
Grief Diaries: Surviving Loss of a Loved One
Grief Diaries: Surviving Loss by Suicide
Grief Diaries: Surviving Loss of Health
Grief Diaries: How to Help the Newly Bereaved
Grief Diaries: Loss by Impaired Driving
Grief Diaries: Through the Eyes of an Eating Disorder
Grief Diaries: Loss by Homicide
Grief Diaries: Loss of a Pregnancy
Grief Diaries: Living with a Brain Injury
Grief Diaries: Hello from Heaven
Grammy Visits From Heaven
Faith, Grief & Pass the Chocolate Pudding

FORTHCOMING TITLES (PARTIAL LIST):
Shattered
Heaven Talks to Children
Color My Soul Whole
Grief Reiki
Grief Diaries: Through the Eyes of a Funeral Director
Grief Diaries: You're Newly Bereaved, Now What?
Grief Diaries: Life After Organ Transplant
Grief Diaries: Raising a Disabled Child
Grief Diaries: Living with Rheumatic Disease
Grief Diaries: Through the Eyes of Cancer
Grief Diaries: Loss of a Client
Grief Diaries: Poetry & Prose and More
Grief Diaries Life After Rape
Grief Diaries: Living with Mental Illness
Grief Diaries: Through the Eyes of D.I.D.
Grief Diaries: Living with PTSD
Grief Diaries: Living with a Brain Injury
Where Have All The Children Gone: A Mother's Journey Through Complicated Grief

ALYBLUE MEDIA

HEALING TOGETHER PROGRAM

Dedicated to raising awareness, and offer comfort and hope in the aftermath of painful experiences, AlyBlue Media's Healing Together Program donates a portion of profits from each title to a national organization serving those in need. The nonprofit recipients are determined by the writers who contribute to book series.

There's a bright future for you at every turn,
even if you miss one.

*

To share your story in a Grief Diaries book, visit
www.griefdiaries.com

Published by AlyBlue Media
Inside every human is a story worth sharing.
www.AlyBlueMedia.com